KETO DIET FOR BEGINNERS

Step-by-step Guide to INTERMITTENT FASTING on a Ketogenic Diet

Loose up to 21ltb with the Ultimate 21-Day Meal Plan with Recipes for rapid weight loss

By

Anastasia Hawkins

Table of Content

Chapter 1: 12
   What is Keto Diet? 12
   Types of Ketosis: 13
      ☐ Fasting Ketosis: 13
      ☐ High Protein Ketosis: 15
      ☐ Cyclic Ketosis: 15
      ☐ Targeted Ketosis: 16
   How much time does it take to enter Ketosis? 16
   Tracking Carbohydrate Intake: 17
   Balance weight loss with Protein Intake: 18
   Tips to Achieving Ketosis: 20
      ☐ Add coconut oil in your diet: 20
      ☐ Engage in Physical Activity: 21
      ☐ Try Fasting: 21
      ☐ Keep the Protein Intake Moderate: 21
      ☐ Go for a Ketone Test: 22
   Perks of Ketosis: 22
      ☐ Weight Loss: 23
      ☐ Fights Acne: 23
      ☐ Great for Heart: 24
      ☐ Efficient Brain functioning: 24

- ☐ Effective for Metabolic Syndrome: 24

Essential Keto Diet Tools for Getting Started: 25

- ☐ Instant Pot: 26
- ☐ Milk Frother: 26
- ☐ Cast Iron Skillet: 26
- ☐ Food Processor: 26
- ☐ Digital Food Scale: 27
- ☐ Griller: 27
- ☐ Air Fryer: 27
- ☐ Silicon Baking Mats: 28

Chapter 2: Keto Do's and Don't's 29

Keto Substitutes; Swapping High Carb Food and Unhealthy Fats 29

- ☐ Swap Flour with Almond Flour: 29
- ☐ Swap Tortillas with Lettuce Leaves: 30
- ☐ Try Cauliflower Rice instead of Plain Rice: 30
- ☐ Replace Regular Coffee with Bulletproof Coffee: 31
- ☐ Swap Milk with Almond Milk: 31
- ☐ Use Fathead Crust for Pizza Crust: 31
- ☐ Veggie Noodles instead of Pasta: 32
- ☐ Swap Vegetable Oil with Coconut Oil: 32

Making Healthier Protein Choices 33

Fresh fruits on the go: 34

- Keto Friendly Sweeteners: 35
  - ☐ Stevia: 36
  - ☐ Sucralose: 36
  - ☐ Xylitol: 37
  - ☐ Monk Fruit Sweetener: 37
  - ☐ Yacon Syrup: 37
- Understanding the Glycemic Index 38
- Stocking up a Keto Refrigerator: 41
  - ☐ Dairy Products: 42
  - ☐ Fruits: 42
  - ☐ Meat and Fish: 43
  - ☐ Vegetables: 43
- Pick Smart, Keto-Friendly Beverages: 44
- Fresh and Frozen Veggies; Go Green: 46
- Foods to Avoid during Ketosis: 48
- Alcoholic Beverages: 49

Chapter 3: Adapting a Ketogenic Lifestyle for a Healthy Living 51

- Understanding Macros in Ketosis: 54
- Guidelines for Dairy, Meat and Vegetables 59
- How does Keto help in Weight Loss; effects on human body: 63
- Steps for Transition into Keto Diet: 66

Part 2-Step by Step Guide To Intermittent Fasting 70

Chapter 4: What Is Intermittent Fasting? 70

    The Science behind Intermittent Fasting; 72

    Benefits of Intermittent Fasting 73

- ☐ Weight Loss: 73
- ☐ Reduces Oxidative Stress: 74
- ☐ Stronger Heart: 74
- ☐ Happier and Healthier Brain: 74

    Autophagy: 75

    How Fasting burns Fat? 76

    Everything runs on Hormones: 78

Chapter 5: Hormones VS Fasting; How does it work? 79

    Role of Insulin in Human Body: 81

    Insulin and Intermittent Fasting: 82

    Meet your Hunger Hormones; Leptin and Ghrelin: 82

    How are both these diets a miracle for burning fat? 84

    The 21 Day Meal Plans: 85

    Week 1: 86

    Day 1: 86

    Monday 86

- ☐ Breakfast; Scrambled Eggs: 86
- ☐ Lunch: Keto No Noodle Chicken Soup: 87
- ☐ Dinner: Keto Carbonara: 88

Day 2: 88

Tuesday: 88

- [ ] Breakfast: Keto Frittata with Fresh Spinach: 88
- [ ] Lunch; Keto Asian Beef Salad: 89
- [ ] Dinner: Baked Salmon with Asparagus: 91

DAY 3: 92

Wednesday: 92

- [ ] Breakfast: 3 Egg Omelet with Spinach, Sausage and Cheese 92
- [ ] BLT Salad: 92
- [ ] Dinner; Keto Pesto Casserole: 93

Day 4: 94

Thursday: 94

- [ ] Breakfast: Keto Cheese Roll Ups: 94
- [ ] Lunch: Keto Caprese Omelet: 95
- [ ] Dinner: Keto Meat Pie 96

Day 5: 97

Friday 97

- [ ] Breakfast: Dairy Free Keto Latte: 97
- [ ] Lunch: Keto Avocado, Bacon and Goat Cheese Salad: 98
- [ ] Dinner: Keto Pizza: 99

Day 6: 100

Friday: 100
- ☐ Breakfast: Mushroom Omelet: 100
- ☐ Lunch: Keto Smoked Salmon: 101
- ☐ Dinner: Keto Asian Cabbage Stir Fry: 101

Day 7: 103

Sunday: 103
- ☐ Breakfast: Keto Pancakes with Whipped Cream and Berries: 103
- ☐ Lunch: Italian Keto Plate: 105
- ☐ Dinner: Keto Tortilla with Ground Beef and Salsa: . 105

Week 2: 106

Day 8: 106

Monday: 106
- ☐ Breakfast: No bread, keto breakfast sandwich: 106
- ☐ Lunch: Keto Tuna Salad with Boiled Eggs: 107
- ☐ Dinner: Keto Hamburger Patties with Tomato Sauce: 108

Day 9: 109

Tuesday: 109
- ☐ Breakfast: Bulletproof Coffee: 109
- ☐ Lunch: Keto roast beef and cheddar plate: 110
- ☐ Dinner: Keto Fried Salmon with Broccoli and Cheese: 110

Day 10: 112

Wednesday: 112

☐ Breakfast: Keto Coconut Porridge: 112

☐ Lunch: Keto shrimp and artichoke plate: 113

☐ Dinner: Keto Chicken Casserole: 114

Day 11: 114

Thursday: 114

☐ Breakfast: Keto Egg Muffins: 114

☐ Lunch: Keto Cauliflower Soup with crumbled pancetta: 115

☐ Dinner: Keto Cheeseburger: 117

Day 12: 117

Friday: 117

☐ Breakfast: Boiled Eggs with Mayonnaise: 117

☐ Lunch: Keto Caesar Salad: 118

☐ Dinner: Fathead Pizza: 118

Day 13: 121

Saturday: 121

☐ Breakfast: Western Omelet Breakfast: 121

☐ Lunch: Keto prosciutto-wrapped asparagus with goat cheese: 122

☐ Dinner: Creamy Keto Fish Casserole: 123

Day 14: 124

Sunday: 124
- ☐ Breakfast: Classic Bacon and Eggs: 124
- ☐ Lunch: Keto Salmon filled Avocados: 124
- ☐ Dinner: Keto Ribeye Steak with oven-roasted vegetables: 126

Week 3 126

Day 15: 126

Monday: 126
- ☐ Breakfast: Keto Avocado Eggs with Bacon Sails: 126
- ☐ Lunch: Diary Free Butter Chicken: 127
- ☐ Dinner: Salad Sandwiches 128

Day 16: 129

Tuesday: 129
- ☐ Breakfast: Keto Tuna Salad with Capers: 129
- ☐ Lunch: Bacon Spinach Frittata: 130
- ☐ Dinner: Low Carb Taco Pie: 131

Day 17: 131

Wednesday: 131
- ☐ Breakfast: Breakfast Tapas: 131
- ☐ Lunch: Keto Turkey with Cream Cheese Sauce: 132
- ☐ Dinner: Chops Marinated in Red Pesto: 134

Day 18: 134

Thursday: 134

- ☐ Breakfast: Fried Eggs: 134
- ☐ Lunch: Bison Meatballs with Zoodles and Chimichurri Sauce: 135
- ☐ Dinner: Keto baked Salmon with Pesto: 136

Day 19: 137

Friday: 137

- ☐ Breakfast: Scrambled Egg with Basil and Butter: 137
- ☐ Lunch: California Turkey and Bacon Wraps with Basil Mayo: 138
- ☐ Dinner: Keto Meatballs: 139

Day 20: 140

Saturday: 140

- ☐ Breakfast: Keto Cauliflower Hash with Eggs and Poblano Peppers: 140
- ☐ Lunch: Blackened Shrimp, Asparagus and Avocado Salad: 141
- ☐ Dinner: Keto Bacon Sushi: 143

Day 21: 144

Sunday: 144

- ☐ Breakfast: Keto Fried Eggs with Kale and Pork: 144
- ☐ Lunch: Salad with Roasted Cauliflower: 145
- ☐ Dinner: Garlicky Lemon Mahi-Mahi: 145

Self-care Tips for Transition in Ketosis Intermittent Fasting: 147

    Important Minerals and Vitamins during Ketosis: 147

How to work out while on Ketogenic Fasting?..................... 149

Chapter 1:

Everyone seems to be appreciating the perks of keto diet these days. The low carb and high-fat eating diet plan is the perfect choice to make if you want your body to burn fat rapidly, like a machine. Due to its ability to help you amazingly with weight loss, keto diet has become one of the best diet plans. It has gathered a lot of popularity and many public figures are seen discussing its benefits too.

What is Keto Diet?

Ketogenic diet, also referred to as Keto diet, is one of the most popular diet plans these days. It is focuses on the amount and type of carbs and fats that you can consume so that your body can burn the stored fat.

Keto diet emphasizes on the production of "ketones" which are small molecules that help in fueling your body's ability to burn fat. Ketones are produced by the human body when you have low carb intake and very moderate amount of protein. Moreover, these molecules are created when your blood sugar (glucose) is in short supply. Thus, low carb and moderate protein intake are two of the easiest ways to boost the production of ketones.

Liver is responsible for ketone creation. It produces ketones through fat and then these molecules serve as a fuel for the human body, especially the brain. Brain consumes a lot of energy and it is one of the most energy consuming organ. As it only runs efficiently through glucose or ketones; thus, the keto diet focuses on the production on ketones instead of glucose.

Therefore, the keto diet runs your body on fat and by burning fat throughout the day, through ketones. As glucose levels become low, the body is able to burn fat rapidly. Through keto diet, human body is able to access the stored fat and burn it swiftly. This is why ketogenic diet is considered ideal for people who are trying to lose weight. If you are facing focus issues, then keto diet can really help in enhancing your focus and productivity. It is going to take some days to put your body in a state of ketosis but once it enters the phase; it gets easier.

Types of Ketosis:

There is no certain, one plan, to put your body into the state of ketosis. There are 4 basic types of ketosis or keto diets and they all tend to serve different people with different purposes. They also vary in the level of ketone production for your body.

- **Fasting Ketosis:**
  Fasting has played a major part in the keto diet and it also has been around for years. A lot of

philosophers have also appreciated the perks of fasting. Scientists and philosophers definitely understood the benefits of fasting way before time but the modern world are now praising its perks too.

The potentials of fasting are incredible and many people opt for fasting ketosis too. As ketosis focuses on low levels of glucose because it increases the fat burning process, fasting can actually help in doing so too. Restricting food intake for a few hours can lower the glucose levels and start accessing the stored fat for producing ketone and utilizing it for energy and regular productivity levels.

Short fasting period won't boost ketone production at all. You certainly need to fast for a longer time span to make sure that ketone production is able to surpass the ketone clearance. It does not mean that ketosis won't happen with short fasts but the ketone production is extremely minor in shorter fasts which won't result in good weight loss outcomes. Detains refer to longer fasts so that the energy levels remain in an equilibrium and no body mass is lost either.

There are different types of ketosis fasting that one can opt for. Intermittent fasting, overnight fasting or alternate day fasting are 3 of the best types of fasting keto diets that one can opt for. However, intermittent fasting is one of the best ways to lose weight. Also, majority of people select it too.

- **High Protein Ketosis:**

    For everyone who is wishing to shred the excessive bod fat; high protein keto diet is the best pick to make. The basic aim of this type of ketosis is to drop the extra fat from the body and not just the weight. A high protein diet helps the body in maintaining the lean body mass which is of great help for people who work out. Furthermore, this type uses the stored fat while you work to enhance weight loss. High protein basically boosts the fat burning effect but keeps the energy and strength maximum at all times.

- **Cyclic Ketosis:**

    Cyclic ketosis is the 3rd type of ketosis or keto diet which is mostly chosen by advanced athletes. As they need a lot of energy during training, this form of ketosis focuses on high carb intake. In cyclic ketosis, athletes are allowed to boost the intake of carbs 2 days before their competition so that their body has glycogen stored in abundance. Cyclic ketosis also promotes muscle power and growth. However, there is one disadvantage of this type of keto; it can lead to a little fat storage as athletes need to take a lot of carbs before their competition. However, if you are able to burn the stored fat afterwards, then you are good to opt for this type of keto diet.

- **Targeted Ketosis:**
Targeted ketosis allows you to have a good intake of carbs but just right before or after your workout sessions. For anyone who exercises on regular basis, targeted keto diet is a great pick to make. However, the intake of carbs is supposed to be extremely moderate so that they are just enough to provide the human body with the required tolerance. This boosts the workout session of athletes and anyone else who loves working out habitually. 30 or 50g of carbohydrate intake is recommended in targeted keto diet as it is suffice to maintaining decent energy levels during workout sessions.

How much time does it take to enter Ketosis?

Many people assume that they need a week or two to enter the state of ketosis. However, this assumption is completely incorrect as the human body, kicks into the phase of ketosis within 2-3 days. Our bodies only store glucose for 2 day usage, in form of glycogen. Thus, as soon as you start your keto diet and lower down your carb intake; your body enters the state of ketosis within a matter of 2 days. However, you need to make sure that you are not taking more than 20g of carbs for these 2-3 days. This way, your body will enter ketosis and will start producing ketones and burning fat swiftly.

Tracking Carbohydrate Intake:

Carbohydrates are the macronutrients present in food which promote weight gain as they exceed in intake limit. This is the major reason due to which carb intake is lowered in ketogenic diet. However, the assumptions that keto diet bans all types of carbs on you, is completely false. Also, there is no specification that you cannot exceed a certain amount of carb intake. What you need to do is monitor your carbohydrate intake. Tracking how much carbs you have taken within a day is very important.

Every individual has their own carb limit and in order to boost the production of ketone, that specific amount of carb, needs to go in the human body. Also, according to keto diet, the carb limit keeps altering on different days. Thus, finding your carb limit is very crucial. A lot of people are able to push their body into the state of ketosis with a slightly higher carb intake, in comparison to others. Likewise, some people are able to produce more ketone when they are taking in less carbs. Therefore, knowing and understanding your body's carb intake is essential.

Now, as per keto, every human body needs a different amount of carb, to produce ketones. However, the there is a specified carb intake limit in ketogenic diet, which can help you achieve the state of ketosis faster. The carb limit in keto is 35grams. Now some people might not notice a huge change through this carb intake and you will certainly notice it on your own. Also, if you are referring to a nutritionist throughout your ketogenic diet plan then he/she will let you know your carb limit. The lowest carb intake allowed during keto diet is 20grams and no less than that. It is important to remember that carbohydrates are an essential element, for running the human body properly.

If you are trying to monitor your carbohydrate intake then you can rely on an app as well. Thanks to the technological advancement for the amazing health apps that we have these days. You can easily keep a track of how much carbs you have consumed within a day. Through this, you will be able to monitor your diet properly and won't exceed the keto carb restriction as well. Moreover, it will boost your ketone production and your body will push into the phase of ketosis swiftly.

Balance weight loss with Protein Intake:

Balancing your weight loss is crucial. Majority of people who diet, lose weight fast but are unable to maintain it healthily. The secret to a proper, balanced weight loss is a good protein intake. With moderate or low consumption of carbohydrates, the body requires something that can provide it with the required energy levels and boost it to carry on with regular chores. This is where the significance of protein intake is highlighted. When protein breaks down, it provides the body with the essential amino acids which are scientifically termed as the building blocks of life. Amino acids play an array of functions in the human body and promote a balance within the internal system. They are important for muscle growth, hormone production, a good metabolic system, strong immunity and creation of important enzymes too. Therefore, protein intake cannot be neglected in any case.

Keto diet definitely emphasizes on low carb and high fat intake but people usually cut down on protein a lot. This is where majority of the dieters go wrong and lose their weight loss balance. If you are going to lose your lean body mass; how will you appear to be stunning and fit? The aim of ketogenic diet is to keep you strong internally while you lose the extra, stored fat. If you are not eating enough protein on a keto diet, your energy will go down the aisle.

The biggest issue for keto dieters is that they don't even realize that they are missing out on protein. They are heavily indulged in their carb and fat intake and calculations that protein intake loses its importance. This not only drains the body from energy but it also tends to sabotage your incredible weight loss goals. Thus, make sure that you are not avoiding your protein intake at all. Every type of keto diet allows you to have healthy protein intake in moderate amounts.

Tips to Achieving Ketosis:

Firstly, ketosis is not unhealthy and has a bunch of health perks. It is a normal, metabolic state which runs on ketones, instead of glucose. Ketone becomes your major source of energy during ketosis and this metabolic state has been proven to be remarkable for weight loss. The key rule to achieving ketosis is to lower your carb intake and boost your healthy fats, keeping your protein intake moderate too. However, there are some additional tips that can help you achieve ketosis and enter that state swiftly.

- **Add coconut oil in your diet:**
  Coconut oil is beneficial for ketosis as it has medium chain triglycerides in it. MCT's are an amazing source of fat which are absorbed rapidly and are utilized by the liver, as a source of energy. A lot of studies suggest that coconut oil can boost the chances of entering the phase of ketosis faster as it enhances ketone production.

- **Engage in Physical Activity:**
  As your carb intake is low, it is important to engage yourself in physical activity, so that ketone production is enhanced. With carb intake low, storage of glycogen is extremely low as well, which means that the body accesses stored fat for energy purposes. It is not essential that you join a gym for physical activity. You can simply indulge in bricking walking for 20-30 minutes daily or you can simply go for a run.

- **Try Fasting:**
  Fasting ketosis is a type of keto diet which is opted by majority of people as it pushes the body into ketosis faster. Intermittent fasting is the best type of fasting ketosis as it boosts the creation of ketones like none other. Short fasts usually don't enhance the level of ketones as much as longer fasts do. Thus, it is recommended that you try the 8 and 16 hour eating window which ensures great levels of ketone production and wonderful weight loss as well.

- **Keep the Protein Intake Moderate:**
  Ditch all the myths about keto diet which suggest you to have a low protein intake. With protein levels going low, your body won't be able to lose weight and even if it does, it won't be a balanced and healthy

weight loss. Protein ensures the production of amino acids which regulates several functions within the human body. Thus, to push yourself into ketosis, you need to lower your carb intake, eat more healthy fats and keep your proteins along as well. Nobody wants to lose their lean body mass and protein will help you, in staying fit and healthy while losing the bad fat.

- **Go for a Ketone Test:**
  Many people doubt that they are not entering the state of ketosis and it might be true. Every individual has their own body type and they need to restrict their carb intake accordingly too. If you think that your body is not responding very well to the keto diet, then you might have to get a keto test done. This will help you in understanding how much more restriction is required, to get your body in the phase of ketosis.

By inculcating these easy 5 tips in your keto diet, you can easily achieve ketosis and boost your ketone production, whilst remaining healthy and energetic too.

Perks of Ketosis:

A lot of people assume that ketosis make a person lethargic and deprives him/her from the basic needs of human body.

However, this assumption, rather myth, is completely false. Ketosis or keto diet has a bunch of health benefits which makes it one of the most appreciated and popular diet plans of all times. It is being praised by celebrities, models and normal people as well. It not only boosts weight loss but ensures a healthy plan of losing the unwanted, stored fat. The major aim is to lower your caloric intake through carbs and keep it moderate through protein and healthy fat intake. The human body is provided with all the healthy items that it needs, in order to stay in shape, while encouraging a healthier lifestyle too. Here are some of the benefits of ketosis and how it is able to provide different advantages to the human body:

- **Weight Loss:**
  We all know that keto diet is incredible for a balanced weight loss. As the stored fat is burned, it ensures a healthier journey towards losing weight and it is easier to maintain as well. This is one of the most popular diets right now, for weight loss.

- **Fights Acne:**
  Ketosis helps in reducing acne as well. There are several reasons for acne and high blood sugar levels are also one of them. As the glucose storage is restricted in ketosis, it aids in reducing acne, promoting a healthier skin. Also, the refined and

processed carbs are one of the biggest reasons for acne. As keto encourages healthy and low intake of carb, the blood sugar level fluctuations are lowered which automatically fights acne, bringing a positive influence of the skin.

- **Great for Heart:**
  If you are able to follow the keto diet in a healthy way, it becomes extremely beneficial for your heart health. Ketosis reduces cholesterol which is the major culprit for cardiac issues. Thus, by stimulating balanced cholesterol levels, ketosis aids in keeping the heart healthier.

- **Efficient Brain functioning:**
  In the light of studies, keto diet is capable of offering neuroprotective advantages. It can provide a shield from various brain diseases like Parkinson's and Alzheimer's. Furthermore, ketosis also helps with sleeping disorders and enhances the quality of sleep overall.

- **Effective for Metabolic Syndrome:**
  Metabolic syndrome links with higher risks for heart diseases and diabetes. It is a group of different symptoms that affects a lot of different organs, rather than just the metabolism. It is going to elevate

your blood pressure, sugar levels, promote obesity and triglycerides. All of these are further going to make you prone towards life endangering diseases. Thus, with the help of ketosis, you are able to put all these symptoms aside. With low carb intake, you are able to control your blood pressure and sugar levels and also lose weight in a healthy way.

There have been massive bad assumptions about keto diet since a long time but through research and various studies, the benefits of ketosis are being unfolded. These are able to unveil the good side of keto diet and how it is able to promote a healthier lifestyle overall. It is not just beneficial for weight loss but is also amazing for blood pressure, diabetes, brain and the human heart.

Essential Keto Diet Tools for Getting Started:

Whether you are a beginner with keto diet or you have been attempting to this diet plan since a long time; some tools are certainly going to be your helping hand along the journey. During ketosis, you have to spend your time in the kitchen more and more as you are responsible for your own meals. Here are some essential tools that are important to get started with keto diet, in your kitchen. These will ensure great fluency while you plan and cook your own meals.

- **Instant Pot:**

  An instant pot is going to help you amazingly with your keto diet meals. From baked goods, hard boiled eggs to soups and roasts, you can make anything in this, within a matter of minutes.

- **Milk Frother:**

  Bulletproof coffee is a go-to item in keto diet, for a lot of people. This tool just makes it easier to make the best ever bulletproof coffee, within minutes. It is considered as a great source of healthy fat, so started your day with it, is going to boost your ketone production. With the help of a good Frother, you are able to get a latte like coffee, right at home.

- **Cast Iron Skillet:**

  Cast iron skillets might seem hard to handle but once you are used to them, you definitely do not want to go back to the others. It is a must have for keto dieters as it is able to cook the best sear steaks ever. You can also bake your burgers in it' so why not invest in one and make your life easier?

- **Food Processor:**

  Whether you are on a keto diet or not, this is one of the most essential tools for every meal ever. A good food processor and blender just tend to make your life easier with cooking whatever you want to. Within minutes you can make some of the best protein shakes, boosting your body energy levels perfectly.

- **Digital Food Scale:**
  When you start keto diet, you do start to monitor your food and your portions. This is why; a digital food scale is an important tool for all keto dieters. It might not seem vital to a lot of people but if you are attempting to ketosis diet plan seriously, then this is a good tool to possess.

- **Griller:**
  A griller is going to cook simply anything and everything. Grilling your meat, so that it stays healthy for you, is one of the best ways to stay on track, while at a keto diet. You can simply make all your protein meals on a griller, ensuring that you are not frying them in tons of oil and are staying on the healthier track. Also, a griller is going to make your meat juicier and much tastier.

- **Air Fryer:**
  The basic key to keto might be large intake of fat but it has to be healthy fat. Thus, an air fryer is going to cook all the meals for you, without a lot of oil. You are going to get a healthy and mummy meal with this

tool and this is definitely an important one to have in your kitchen.

- **Silicon Baking Mats:**

These baking mats are a blessing in your kitchen as they are going to make the best ever keto pizzas for you. Your perfect keto cookies and pretzels are going to be baked to perfection with these silicon mats. Thus, make sure that you invest in these as most of the times; you will be baking your meals.

Chapter 2: Keto Do's and Don't's

Ketogenic diet is more of a trend these days as it helps people in attaining the dramatic weight loss that everyone wishes for these days. However, the good side to keto is that the dramatic weight loss is also healthy. It focuses on providing your body with all the essentials it needs, cutting down on the elements that the body can actually survive without, in a good way. In this chapter, we will be discussing all the dos and don'ts of keto diet in detail, to understand the best way to ketosis.

Keto Substitutes; Swapping High Carb Food and Unhealthy Fats

Ketosis is all about low carb intake and healthy fat and protein intake. Therefore, you have to swap a lot of high carb food items with low carb ones, ensuring that your body enters the state of ketosis swiftly. If you know of all the good substitutes, then you won't feel a lot of difference in your overall diet plan at all. Many people ditch the keto diet because they have no idea about the healthier and good food substitutes that can be eaten during ketosis.

- **Swap Flour with Almond Flour:**
  Flour is the basic ingredient to several delicious meals. It is important for baking and cooking both. Thus, ditching it completely is a little hard. For the

sake of low carb diet, you can replace flour with almond flour. Almond flour has fewer carbs than regular flour and has more protein and fat in it. Thus, it is a perfect keto substitute.

- **Swap Tortillas with Lettuce Leaves:**
Ditch the tortillas and opt for lettuce leaves. Tacos are all carbs, thus leaving them out of your keto diet is essential. However, you can hold all your ingredients or delicious taco mixture together, with the help of lettuce leaves. It might not sound appealing at all but it actually is. Once you try it on your own, you will love it.

- **Try Cauliflower Rice instead of Plain Rice:**
Plain or regular white rice are extremely high in carbs and during keto, you have to leave them out of your meals. However, you can opt for cauliflower rice. They look the same as regular rice and are going to taste a lot like them too. The only difference that you might feel is going to be their texture. Cauliflower rice is a little harder than regular ones. Even when you cook them for a good time span, the hardness does remain.

- **Replace Regular Coffee with Bulletproof Coffee:**
Many people ditch their coffee and no sooner, they ditch keto diet. Caffeine is addictive and anyone who has been a coffee lover since years won't be able to leave it out of the diet. Thus, you can replace your coffee with bulletproof coffee as it boosts the ketone creation and ensures that your metabolic state goes into ketosis. Bulletproof coffee is very easy to make and has the same taste too or even a little better than the regular coffee.

- **Swap Milk with Almond Milk:**
Milk is higher in carb but almond milk is perfect when it comes to carb intake. It has lower amount of carbs and makes a wonderful substitute for anyone who loves drinking milk. Almond milk is a bit thinner than regular milk but you don't really notice the difference much. The texture is definitely less creamy but it is a good replacement as it tastes good too.

- **Use Fathead Crust for Pizza Crust:**
Who said you cannot have pizza while on a keto diet? Whoever did, simply did not know of this substitute. Keto dieters use fathead crust for pizza crust and make sure that they can have a good and tasty pizza

often. If you are a pizza lover, this is definitely good news for you. You don't have to leave the love of your life behind to follow keto diet. Just use fathead crust and you are good to go.

- **Veggie Noodles instead of Pasta:**
Pasta is the core ingredient for so many dishes and missing out on it is a little hard. However, veggie noodles help you in this difficult situation. You can simply swap pasta with veggie noodles and enjoy your meals. The biggest perk of these noodles is that they are very simple to make and require very little time to cook, in comparison with pasta.

- **Swap Vegetable Oil with Coconut Oil:**
Vegetable oil is extremely high in carbs and is not an option in keto diet. This is why swapping vegetable oil with coconut oil is a smarter choice to make. It has healthier fat and less carbs which is the perfect combo for keto dieters. The saturated fat in coconut oil is extremely beneficial as it is going to boost your energy levels amazingly. With low carb intake, you can run out of energy easily. Thus coconut oil will fuel it up for you.

So you see? There are a lot of different food substitutes for anyone who wants to opt for keto diet and is afraid of excluding a lot of food items from their life. Just opt for good substitutes and you are fine to go with ketosis.

Making Healthier Protein Choices

Protein carries out a number of essential functions in the human body, due to which, it holds immense importance overall. It is extremely vital for every individual to have an adequate intake of protein so that they can enhance their healthy lifestyle. Protein is not only incredibly useful for muscle growth and repair but is extremely essential for hormone and enzyme creation as well. Furthermore, it helps in maintaining your skin, hair and several internal organs.

Considering the fact that protein is an essential asset for every human, its intake, during keto diet, remains moderate. A lot of people assume that their protein intake has to be tremendously low during ketosis but that is incorrect. Without proper protein intake, you will feel drained and your energy levels will remain low. Thus, it is recommended that every keto dieter must include 1.2 or 1.7 grams of protein in their diet. For some people, an intake of up to 2 grams is also fine. However, no more than 2g of protein intake is entertained in ketogenic.

On the other hand, people who are indulging in keto diet for therapeutic reasons might have to lower down their protein intake to 1gram only. However, the protein portions are best settled by a nutritionist for a diet. As the intake is highly dependent on the body weight, it is important that one selects their amount of intake under medical supervision. This will ensure a healthier you!

Fresh fruits on the go:

Fruits are a vital part of everybody's diet but many of them are restricted during ketosis. Why? This is because the keto style diet focuses on low carb intake and most of the fruits are high in carbs. This is the major reason due to which they are naturally sweet. However, there are also of fruits which are still allowed during the keto diet and they are easier to carry around with you too.

Most of the fruits are extremely high in carbs. For instance, a banana has 25grams of carbs in it. If you eat a banana, you are exceeding your carb intake limit during ketosis. Thus, a lot of fruits are not allowed during keto diet.

While you are on ketogenic diet, you are only going to be allowed to carry the following fruits with you:

- **Blackberries**: half cup of blackberries (70g) provides you with just 4 grams of carbs

- **Raspberries:** Half cup of raspberries (60g) offers 3 grams of carbs

- **Strawberries:** 8 medium sized strawberries (100g) have 6 grams of carbs

- **Blueberries:** Half cup of blueberries (75g) provides you with 9 grams of carbs

- **Plum:** A medium sized plum (65g) provides you with 7 grams of carbs.

These are the only fruits that are allowed during ketosis as they provide you with lesser carbs but more energy. Berries are renowned for the endless perks that they have to offer and are considered extremely healthy too. It is best to keep half cup of any of these berries or a medium sized plum you, while you go out. If you feel a sudden craving, you can snack with these fruits. It is always best if you take fresh fruits but if you don't have an option to do so, it is best to carry one along with you, from home. Also, these fruits are extremely fulfilling and give you a satisfied feeling as well which means that you won't feel the urge to snack anytime sooner after having these.

Keto Friendly Sweeteners:

By now, everyone understands and knows the items that have to be cut down during a ketogenic diet. Anything that is high in carbs, or is processed, is not allowed in this popular diet plan. Desserts and meaningless snacks are the foremost items that get cut down during ketosis and if you have a sweet tooth, then this might be the harshest thing to attempt to. However, there is still a savior that can provide you with a bit of sweet tooth, without disrupting your diet restrictions. Here are the top 5 keto friendly sweeteners which are extremely low in carbs and won't let you exceed your carb intake limit at all.

- **Stevia:**

    Stevia is an all-natural sweetener and is one of the best keto friendly sweeteners to look forward to. It is popular because it has almost "no calories" included. Moreover, studies portray that stevia does help in lowering glucose which obviously boost ketone production and aid in ketosis. Also, while you replace sugar with stevia, you must know that stevia has a stronger taste. You just need a teaspoon of stevia for substituting a cup of regular white sugar.

- **Sucralose:**

    This is an artificial sweetener but is a great keto friendly one too. Sucralose is not metabolized which means that it passes through the body, without offering any carbs or calories. Splenda is one of the best sucralose based keto friendly sweetener available in the market these days and is also one of the most used ones. It is recommended that you keep sucralose in colder temperatures as keeping it in hot and humid places can promote production of harmful compounds in it.

- **Xylitol:**
  Xylitol is commonly found in sugar free chewing gums and candies and is a sugar alcohol, keto friendly sweetener. With just 3 calories per one gram, xylitol offers you the same taste as regular sugar. With one teaspoon of this sweetener added to any of your meal, you are only consuming 4grams of carbs which is perfect for a keto dieter.

- **Monk Fruit Sweetener:**
  This sweetener is derived naturally from the monk fruit which is found in South China. It has sugary compounds in it naturally which provide you with the required sweetness. The best part about monk fruit sweetener is that it has no carbs or calories in it and is almost as sweet as regular sugar or slightly a bit more.

- **Yacon Syrup:**
  Yacon syrup is another all-natural keto friendly sweetener and is found in the Yacon plant which is native to South America. This sweetener has almost 20 calories per tablespoon which might be a lot for a keto dieter. There is obviously something else that

you are going to add to your meal and you don't want to exceed your limit for carb or calorie intake too. Thus, it is recommended that one uses Yacon syrup a little less. Other sweeteners have fewer calories and carbs in them, which is why, they are used more widely.

You don't have to completely ditch your desserts while on ketosis. You can easily carry your keto diet on and make smart substitutes so that your low carb intake remains constant. For instance, you can replace flour with almond flour and likewise, you can use one of the above mentioned sweeteners to bake any keto cookie that you are craving.

Understanding the Glycemic Index

Ketogenic diet is highly connected with the glycemic index and before you begin your journey towards ketosis, it is crucial that you understand this index. It will help you enter the state of ketosis in a much better way.

So what is the glycemic index? It basically helps you in measuring the rate on which the foods consumed; raise your blood sugar levels. The foods you consume are ranked on a scale from 0 to 100 and glucose is given the value of 100. Simpler carbs are the ones that burn faster and thus, they are on the higher edge of the glycemic index scale. The human body usually craves these types of carbs when glucose levels fall low in the body. The simple carbs provide you with instant energy and therefore, they are craved more. On the contrary, complex carbs which are slow to burn are on the lower edge of the glycemic index scale. These carbs keep your blood sugar levels moderate.

To understand the index, you must know about the simpler and complex carbs. Here are some simple carbs which burn faster:

- Juice
- White bread
- Chips
- Rice cakes
- Dried fruits
- Candy
- Sweeteners

Here is a list of complex carbs which burn slowly:

- Nuts
- Whole grains
- Non-starchy vegetables
- Beans
- Legumes
- Fruits

Getting a glycemic index for the common foods that you eat is going to help you understand your carbohydrate intake. It will further help you eliminate the high carb foods and include the low carb ones. Here are some examples of common carb food and their number of the GI scale:

- Cornflakes (92 GI scale)-extremely high
- Apple (40 GI scale)-low
- Oatmeal (55 GI scale)-medium
- Banana (51 GI scale)-medium
- Baked Potato (82 GI scale)-very high

Once you start checking the glycemic index scale of your common food items, you will notice that foods like pasta and chips rank medium on the GI scale. Foods with a medium GI scale are easily absorbed by the body. So if you have been working out a lot or have just done a jog or run, then eating these foods won't affect you negatively. However, you need to remember that the key to success in ketosis is moderation. Don't exceed the intake restrictions that come with the keto diet, elsewise, your body won't produce a lot of ketone.

If you are not a workout person and would prefer bringing in the required changes in your diet, then you need to opt for foods that rank low on the GI scale. These are foods like:

- Hummus (10 GI Scale)-extremely low

- Almonds (0 GI scale)

- Lentils (29 GI Scale)-low

These foods are low in carbs and are metabolized gradually but are able to provide you with the much needed energy boost. So this is how glycemic index works and helps you in measuring your keto diet intake properly. By including smart cards in your diet, considering their GI scale, you can easily manage eating smart which is the essence of ketosis.

Stocking up a Keto Refrigerator:

A stocked up pantry and fridge are the keys to success in keto diet. You will have to swap a lot of foods for different, low carb option foods and this will require a proper stock up of your refrigerator. Therefore, here is what you need to stock up a keto fridge with. Before you begin your journey of ketosis, it is important that you pay attention to whatever is lying in your pantry and update it according to the rules of keto. It will help you in the long run as you won't have the foods that are not allowed, within your reach. Therefore, stocking up your pantry and fridge, according to the restriction of ketosis is a major step towards a successful and healthy diet plan.

Here are some basic foods that you would want to stock up before starting a keto diet:

- **Dairy Products:**

    While following a keto diet, milk and yogurt don't really fit in the diet plan. This is because these two items are naturally sweet and high in carbs. The typical limit of a keto diet, carb intake, is 20-30 grams. If your yogurt or milk products consume 6-13 grams just for breakfast or any other meal; then you merely have any carb intake left for the remaining meals. But ketosis also understands the need of dairy products and yogurt is a great essentiality in meals these days. However, you can switch to YQ yogurt which has 2 grams of carbs only. You can also find keto friendly milk options in grocery stores these days but they don't taste really great. Thus, think before you leap for those options.

- **Fruits:**

    Keto does not allow a large fruit variety and this might be a bummer for most fruit lovers. Many people ditch the ketogenic style diet plan because it doesn't offer an array of fruits. Almost all the fruits are restricted in keto apart from the berries. You can have strawberries, blackberries, raspberries and blueberries too. Stock them in your fridge and snack on them to stay healthy and kill the timeless cravings too. You can also have a medium sized plum.

- **Meat and Fish:**

    A lot of people ditch the keto diet because they assume that it restricts protein intake. However, this myth is completely wrong. Protein intake is crucial for humans and it is not restricted in this diet plan at all. However, you are motivated to make smart protein choices and pick foods that don't bombard you with calories. You can have protein that is meat and fish, until and unless you make smart options and portions. Also, make sure that you do know their value on the GI scale as it will help you, to stay in the state of ketosis.

- **Vegetables:**

    Anti-inflammation foods are extremely crucial while you are on a keto diet and vegetables are the key to it. However, you need to make sure that the vegetables you stock up in your refrigerator are all low in carbs. For example, lettuce, spinach, celery, mushrooms, radishes, cucumber, eggplant, tomatoes, zucchini, kale, peppers and cauliflower are some of the best low carb vegetables. These provide you with 1-4 grams of carbs per serving. Thus, stock up on these while you are shopping for your keto meal plan.

You obviously need to put the sugary and processed food items out of your pantry. They have no space in a keto friendly fridge at all. Thus, make smarter choices and update your pantry according to the rules of ketosis, so that your body produces ketones at its best.

Pick Smart, Keto-Friendly Beverages:

Beverages have tons of sugar and carbs in them and sadly, they are the hardest to quit on. If you are a milkshake or fresh juice lover, then you will have to make very wise choices while being on keto diet. As a lot of fruits are not allowed during ketosis, making smarter picks is going to be helpful in the long run. The major element of focus is to keep your beverages as low as zero calories so that your low carb intake is not hindered by them. If you consume tons of carbs and calories through your beverages, your carb intake will boost throughout the day. This won't let your body stay in the phase of ketosis and ketone production will diminish. Therefore, pick smart and keto-friendly beverages if you are looking for some healthy choices. Here is list of keto friendly beverages that you can include in your overall plan:

- **Water:** To begin with, hydration is the key to success during ketosis. You need to make sure that you are well hydrated and water is the most important beverage to keep up with. Drink a lot of water (at least 8 glasses per day) for staying hydrated. Whether you are on ketosis or not; this is the most basic beverage that every individual needs.

- **Coffee and Tea:** Bulletproof coffee is the best beverage for caffeine addicted people in keto diet. You are also allowed to sip on tea but keeping the intake minimum is the best. Also, don't add any sugar to either you cup of coffee or tea. Moreover, drinking these two beverages from fancy restaurants is not going to be of any help as they do add sugar elements in it. Thus, make it at home so that you stay in control of what you drink.

- **Keto Smoothies:** For people who love milkshakes or smoothies, you can swap the sugar ones with keto friendly ones. There are a lot of delicious keto smoothies that are low in calories and carbs and provide you with the same, smoothie feeling as regular one. The key to a keto friendly smoothie is that your produce needs to be low in carbs. Opt for spinach, berries, low carb milk, egg yolks and high fat yogurt to stay on the right path.

- **Alcohol:** Yes, you need to avoid alcohol as much as you can while on a keto diet. However, if you do feel the intense urge of it sometimes, then you can opt for keto friendly options here as well. Light beet, had liquor and unsweetened wines are three of the best options for keto alcohol. Make sure that you keep the intake extremely moderate because it can create havoc in your body and is also very poisonous.

Fresh and Frozen Veggies; Go Green:

A healthy, low carb keto diet is set around vegetables. However, there are some veggies which are high in carbs and are naturally sweet too. Thus, making a wise decision about which vegetables need to be ditched is a bit difficult. Before you choose the vegetables that you can consume during ketosis, it is important that you keep in mind that your daily carb limit is 30 grams. Therefore, keeping your nutrients high and your carbs low, you need to make choices that will help you in the long run, while keeping you healthy and strong too.

There are various ways through which you can include vegetables in your diet. Some people prefer salads and some love making delicious dishes out of them. Either ways, you need to make sure that you are well-aware of the carbs that your vegetables are offering. Here are some of the most low carb vegetables that are recommended during ketosis. Also, there are different ways and styles in which a meal can be planned with these. There is not much vegetable restriction in ketosis and you can enjoy some of the best ones during this diet plan.

- Broccoli has 2.85g carbs in 100g
- Radish has 3.5g carbs in 100g
- Celery has 2.97g carbs in 100g
- Asparagus has 3.88g carbs in 100g
- Olives have 6g carbs in 100g
- Cauliflower has 4.97g carbs in 100g
- Green Beans have 6.97g carbs in 10g
- Eggplant has 5.88g carbs in 100g
- Bamboo shoots have 5.2g carbs in 100g
- Kale has 8.75g carbs in 100g
- Turnips have 6.43g carbs in 100g
- Spinach has 3.63g carbs in 100g
- Zucchini has 3.11g carbs in 100g
- Bok Choi has 2.18g carbs in 100g
- Bell Pepper has 4.6g carbs in 100g
- Cabbage has 6.1g carbs in 100g
- Avocado has 8.6g carbs in 100g
- Cucumber has 3.63g carbs in 100g
- Pumpkin has 7g carbs in 100g

These are 20 vegetables which are low in carb and are extremely beneficial for overall health too. You can get these fresh and frozen both and can prepare wonderful meals with them as well. Also, make sure that if you are planning to eat any other vegetable to your keto diet, then you must know its carb value. If you are mixing different vegetables for a salad, then do weigh them and calculate their total carb value before you gulp it down. Calculating your carb intake is the key to ketosis and will help your body in ketone production as well. Make sure that you do to exceed the limit of 20-30g of carbs at all.

Foods to Avoid during Ketosis:

Now that you have various options for what you can eat during ketosis and what food substitutes you have during this diet plan, it is now time to have a look at the foods that you must avoid. It is best to understand that avoiding these foods is going to help you in ketone production. Here is a list of things that you will have to cut off from while you are following a keto diet:

- Bread
- Rice
- Candy
- Pasta

- Sodas
- Beers
- Juices

- Fruits (apart from berries)
- Chocolates (sweets)
- Potatoes
- Nuts (they are best to avoid but if you do feel like having some; keep the intake low and extremely moderate as they are high in carbs)
- Dairy: High fat dairy is great to consume while on keto diet but it is best to avoid drinking milk as one glass of milk has around 15 carbs. Also avoid café latte. You can obviously add a little milk in your coffee and tea but make sure that you don't add a lot. Also, avoid low fat yogurts by all means and try to use their substitutes instead.

This might seem like a lot of food items but considering the food substitutes mentioned above; you still have a lot of options to choose from. Go ahead and make wise choices so that your body can stay in the state of ketosis for a long period of time.

Alcoholic Beverages:

It is not impossible to have alcohol while on keto. Yes, the intake needs to be extremely moderate but that does not mean that you have to restrict it for a lifetime. A rough estimate is that alcohol has around 7 calories per gram and consuming it in large amounts is definitely going to create a mess with your ketosis.

It is quite obvious that alcoholic drinks like beers and sweet cocktails are extremely high in carbs and can immediately pull your body out from the process of ketosis. They stop the ketone production as the body is provided with immense amount of glucose right away.

This is why it is recommended that alcoholic beverages must be kept moderate in consumption. Make sure that you don't drink it on weekly or daily basis. If you are a spirit drinker and hit on a glass of wine after weeks, then your ketosis is not getting disturbed. However, if you drink too often then your body won't ever be able to achieve a stable state of ketosis. Drinking too much is going to slow down your fat burning process and it will only disrupt your ketosis journey. If you are seriously indulged in keto diet then staying away from alcohol is the best. A little intake in a month is fine and won't hurt you or your efforts. You just need to have control and avoid it every weekend.

Chapter 3: Adapting a Ketogenic Lifestyle for a Healthy Living

Invented in the 1920's, the keto eating style was not much heard of, until two years back. In 2017, ketogenic diet was all over the internet and the hype was real. Nobody really thought that within two years, it will become one of the best diet plans and a healthy lifestyle as well. Majority of people have adapted to ketosis as a lifestyle and not just a diet plan to follow for some weeks. The appreciation that ketogenic diet has received over a little time span is literally mind boggling. However, many people still believe that ketosis is not a great "lifestyle" to opt for. Yes, it is one of the best diet plans but not a complete lifestyle.

The reality is that ketosis is now becoming a lifestyle. People have adapted to it as it allows them to make healthier choices and stay in control of what they eat, along with having knowledge about the choices they are making. Ketosis does add up to one's knowledge immensely. It makes you realize what is healthy for you and what foods are not really offering you much, instead of calories and carbs. Here are some reasons why adapting to a ketogenic lifestyle is going to lead you towards a healthier living.

- **High energy Levels:**

Ditch the myth that says; "ketosis lowers your energy levels." It does not! If you make smart and wise choices while you are on keto, your energy levels are actually boosted. It produces a lot more energy than glucose does and also balances your blood sugar levels which prevent diabetes. Thus, adapting to a keto lifestyle will keep you safe from the adverse effects of glucose but provide you with the benefits of ketone.

- **Great Sexual Activity:**

Many people don't feel the "drive" for having sexual activity with their partners. This behavior is not normal at all and it might be due to your sugar levels or an imbalance in hormones. When you adapt to a keto lifestyle, you basically bring a wonderful equilibrium within your body. Your hormones and enzyme creation and balance gets excellent which help you feel the "mood" whenever your partner wants. A sexual drive is very important to run a good relationship and if you don't feel the urge to make out with your partner then you are too unhealthy from within. However, you can easily fix it with ketosis.

- **No more Meaningless Cravings:**

A keto lifestyle is amazing to adapt as your timeless cravings are simply finished with it. You don't feel the urge to eat timelessly. As you are eating meaningful food that is satisfying and is also providing you with sufficient energy; one does not feel the urge to snack without a reason.

- **Great Brain Function:**

When you adapt a ketogenic lifestyle, you notice that your brain functions really well. You are going to feel more creative and productive. According to studies, ketone is able to fulfill 70% of the brain's needs. Comparing it with glucose, ketones are much better in running the human brain efficiently. As the diet focuses on good fats, which are extremely vital for the brain, this lifestyle offers you a clear and focused mind.

- **Good Sleeping Patterns:**

Ketosis balances your hormones and brings clarity in your mind along with a healthy metabolism which are all, 3 most important aspects for a good sleep. If you have been facing sleep issues then you can adapt a ketogenic lifestyle and you will be blessed with a wonderful sleeping pattern that sets all of your sleeplessness right.

A lot of people choose ketogenic diet for weight loss and don't adapt it as a complete lifestyle. However, once you step in this diet plan, making huge changes in your lifestyle; you do come to realize that keto has a lot more to offer. It has endless perks and it boosts your health in a lot of positive ways. If you are deciding to adapt a ketogenic lifestyle then it is a really good decision to make but it is always best that you discuss it with your nutritionist first.

Understanding Macros in Ketosis:

We have discussed low carbs and healthy fats till now. However, the most essential aspect to consider are the macros as understanding them is going to make your diet plan successful. The best way to understand macros is to break them down individually and then understand how they have to be calculated. Proteins, fats and carbs; all have different macros but combining them all is what is going to help you in pushing your body into ketosis.

First of all, you need to understand what macros are? They are the essential nutrients that the human body requires in order to sustain a good and efficient metabolism system. There are 5 macros according to science:

- Proteins
- Carbohydrates
- Fats
- Water

- Fiber

Although these 5 macros are considered important; the most essential ones are proteins, fats and carbohydrates. These are the key macros of ketosis and a balance between them is extremely crucial for overall health. According to studies, immense reduction or increase in any of these macros, can lead to heart troubles, obesity and much more.

Now, once you understand what macros are; it is time to look at macros from the ketosis point of view. The keto macros are the macronutrients of a ketogenic diet. Here is a ratio of the macros in keto:

- 5-10% caloric intake from carbohydrates
- 15-20% calories from protein
- 60-75% caloric intake from healthy fats

This macro ratio is quite different from the one that people are commonly used to and it is the major reason due to which people are unable to follow ketosis. However, we all know, by now that ketosis works in this manner and even though it is very different from the regular dieting plans; it actually works and is healthy too.

Now we step up to calculating macros in keto. There are different ways in which you can monitor your macros while on ketosis and we are going to discuss them in detail here.

- **Net Carbs:**

    Calculating net carbs is easy; you have to know the total amount of carbs and sinus the number of fiber from it. Calculation of net carbs is vital in ketogenic diet because the body produces glucose through them. Also, fiber has no connection with glucose so you can easily load up on it. Keep in mind that you daily net carb intake restriction in 30g and it must not be exceeded while on ketosis. Also, the most optimal limit is 20g. 30g is the upper limit and a little extension from it is going to kick your body out of ketosis.

- **Proteins:**

    Once you have calculated your net carbs; it is time to move on to the proteins. The protein intake on a ketogenic diet is dependent upon your purpose. Are you following the keto diet for weight loss or for muscle building? For gaining muscles, you need almost 1.5-2.5g of proteins. If you are not following the keto diet for muscle building process, then you can use the following formula to generate your daily intake:

- Start by calculating your body fat through this formula: (the example provided is for an individual who weighs 160 pounds with a body fat percentage of 20%):

    160 pounds x 0.20 (20 %) = 32 pounds of body fat

- Now you need to subtract your body fat percentage from 100 so that you get your lean muscle mass percentage:

    100 - 20 percent (body fat) = 80% of muscle mass

- The next step is to divide the muscle mass by 100 to get the decimal for your muscle weight:

    80 / 100 = 0.80

- Now finally, you need to multiply this decimal by total weight to calculate total lean mass weight:

    160 (pounds) x 0.80 = 128 of lean mass

- The last step is to calculate your daily protein intake by multiplying your muscle mass by gram of protein. The formula for it is:

> 128 pounds (of muscle mass) x 0.7-1 grams (protein per pound of muscle mass) = 89-128 grams of protein

You can easily calculate your protein intake through these steps, according to your own body fat and muscle mass etc.

- **Lastly, you need to calculate the fats:**

    Once your net carb and protein intake has been calculated, the last step is to define your fats. You need a rough estimate of how much fat you need. This, yet again, depends on your purpose; are you trying to lose weight or gain it? A keto calculator is the best tool to calculate your fat intake as it provides you with your personal fat intake limit.

Calculating macros is time consuming but it is the essence of ketosis. Once you are aware of the amount of macros you are taking in, on daily basis, your keto diet stays on track. It will seem boring and toting in the beginning but once you start doing it regularly; you will get by just fine. All you need is a reliable website where you can get the exact ratio of nutrients of different foods that you plan to eat. Making a chart of all of them beforehand is really helpful in the long run.

Guidelines for Dairy, Meat and Vegetables

Ketosis is extremely restrictive and by now, it is quite clear to all the readers, isn't it? In this section, we will be dividing the guidelines for dairy, meat and vegetables separately so that they are easier to understand.

- **Dairy:**

    As a keto dieter, here are some healthy fat dairy products that are okay to include in your diet.

    First of all, butter is the best healthy fat source to rely upon and it is important to include in your ketogenic diet. Butter has absolutely no carbs and offers you around 11g of fat per one tablespoon which is sufficient to provide the needed energy to the body.

    Next up, hard cheeses are another great source of dairy products during ketosis. Parmesan is safe to use during keto and a tablespoon or two is okay to consume. Avoiding semi hard and soft cheese is best during ketosis. However, there are still some soft cheeses that can be considered in a keto diet. Brie Cheese is a great example of soft cheese which has less than 1g of carbs per ounce.

    Whipping cream is a great dairy product to include me your ketogenic diet. Yes, you need to avoid milk by all means because it has a lot of calories and carbs. Adding a bit of milk in tea or coffee is fine but consuming large amount of milk, as it is, is highly restricted. Whipping cream is high in fat and low in carbs and is a definite safe dairy product to use in keto diet.

Dairy products like sour cream, cottage cheese, cream cheese and Greek yogurt are totally allowed during ketosis. A little bit of cream cheese is safe to use. However, over usage is not recommended. Just a tiny bit of cream cheese spread out on your bagel is fine. Items like Greek Yogurt and sour cream or cottage cheese are yet again, keto friendly. Keeping your carb content in check, these three dairy products can be consumed without any worries. Just make sure that you don't cross your keto limit.

- **Veggies:**

Vegetables are primarily composed of carbs and are the ultimate source of low carb intake, during ketosis. However, a lot of veggies are naturally sweet which showcase the presence of high amount of carbs in them, naturally. This is why; you need to know which vegetables are allowed during keto and which ones are restricted.

Vegetables which have a net carb of less than 5g can be eaten freely. You can add a little butter or make a quick sauce with them to create something delicious for yourself. Veggies like zucchini, spinach, kale and asparagus are best keto friendly vegetables as they are hard to consume in larger amounts.

You can definitely include vegetables which are higher than 5g net carb but you will have to keep a good calculation of your carb intake. For example, bell peppers are slightly higher in carb value, thus it is best to use them in really little amount. This will help you remain within the carb restriction so that your body does not step out of the ketosis process.

Similarly, tomatoes are on the higher edge of carbs as they are naturally sweet. You can certainly add them to your meals but you will have to be very careful about them. Also remember that the best carb intake restriction is 20g. This pushes your body to produce ketone faster. However, you are allowed to push the limit till 30g only. It is best if you stay on the 20g limit on most days so that your purpose can be achieved swiftly.

Here are two easy rules to help you understand which veggies are best to eat during ketosis:

- Veggies with leaves are the most keto friendly vegetables to opt for.

- Also remember that green veggies are relatively lower in carbs than other vegetables. Thus relying on them the most is going to keep you safer. They also tend to give a more satisfying feeling to your stomach which kills the meaningless cravings and timeless hunger.

- **Meat:**

Protein intake has always been a subject of argument in ketosis. A lot of people believe the myth that protein intake is highly restricted in ketosis but that is not the case. You need to keep the protein intake moderate, not even low. Protein is responsible for endless functions in the human body and that is why, it is important to have a good, moderate amount of it. To eradicate the confusion for meat lovers, here are the meat sources which are allowed during ketosis. You just need to keep your meat intake moderate and everything works just fine.

- Fish is allowed in ketosis. Moreover, fatter fishes preferred. Fish like salmon, cod, flounder, snapper, tuna and trout are all allowed.

- Beef is also allowed during keto diet. Roasts, stew meat, steaks and ground beefs; you can have them all in moderate portions.

- Pork is also not restricted during ketogenic. Yet again, sticking with fattier cuts is better and avoids adding sugar to it.

- Other meat sources like turkey, lamb, veal and goat are also allowed.

- In poultry, you can rely on chicken, quail, duck and other wild animals too.

The meat restriction is not large (comparing it to the carb limitations). However, you need to watch out for the portions to eat. The amount of meat you take must remain adequate as you don't want to ruin the ketone production process. Thus, low carb and medium protein intake with a high fat intake is all that needs to be followed during ketosis.

How does Keto help in Weight Loss; effects on human body:

Keto diet has embraced a lot of appreciation and praise due to its weight loss benefits. This high fat and low carb diet has proven to be extremely healthy overall. It actually makes your body burn fat, like a machine which is why;

public figures are also highly appreciative of it. But the question is how does ketosis boost weight loss? Here is a detailed insight to the process of ketosis and weight loss.

Ketosis is considered abnormal by some people. Despite the fact that it has been approved by a lot of nutritionists and doctors; a lot of people still disapprove of it. The misconceptions are all due to the myths that have been spread around about the ketogenic diet.

Ketogenic diet is a normal diet plan and the process of ketosis is a normal, metabolic function. The rule is to lower the blood sugar levels so that the body accesses the stored, extra fat to produce energy. Once your body does not have glucose, it is automatically going to rely on the stored fat. Also, it is important to understand that carbs create glucose and once you start taking a low carb diet, you will be able to lower the glucose levels as well. Thus, your body is going to create the fuel through fats, instead of carbs, that is glucose.

The process of creating fuel through fat is known as ketosis and once your body enters this state, it becomes extremely efficient in burning the unwanted fat. Also, as glucose levels are low during ketogenic diet, your body attains a lot of other health benefits as well.

This is how your body burns fat rapidly during ketosis, providing you with intense and amazing weight loss outcomes. Ketogenic diet is not just helpful for weight loss but also aids in boosting your overall health in positive ways. Unlike all the other diet plans, which focus on cutting down your caloric intake, keto emphasis on putting your body in a natural metabolic state, that is ketosis. The only factor that makes this diet plan doubtful is that this nature of metabolism is not talked about a lot. With your body producing ketones regularly, your body will burn the stored fat swiftly which will result in great weight loss.

Now, the query arises; how does ketosis affect the human body?

The truth is that ketogenic diet is healthy for almost everyone. However, one needs to accept that this diet plan is totally different from the ones that we usually try. Thus, your body is definitely going to react a little to the new process. The side effects are termed as "keto flu" during which, one might experience extreme hunger, low energy levels, bad sleeping pattern and a little nauseous as well. However, this phase does not last longer than 2-3 days. This is the time required by the human body to enter the phase of ketosis. Once you have entered it, you are hardly going to have any adverse side effects.

Moreover, you need to start limiting your caloric and carb intake gradually. The most common mistake that keto dieters make is that they tend to start cutting off everything from their diet, all at once. This is where the issue arises. The human body will react extremely negative when you will restrict everything right away. You need to start gradually.

Steps for Transition into Keto Diet:

Adaptation of ketosis can be tough and you will need time to adjust to the changes. It is normal and everyone faces troubles in adapting to any new dietary plan. However, here are some steps to help you in transiting into ketogenic diet plan perfectly. Just remember that it does require time and you will have to give yourself a little space to adjust to the restrictions. It won't happen overnight to don't be disheartened and stay motivated!

- **Gain Knowledge:**

   The most basic mistake that a lot of keto dieters make is that they don't gain enough knowledge, before starting the diet itself. Therefore, the most important step is to gain knowledge and learn the small differences that make a huge difference. Understand what keto friendly foods are what foods are not meant for ketosis at all. For example, a lot of apple does not eat an apple because it has a lot of carbs. However, if you have a medium or a small sized apple, then you are good to have it. As long as it remains within your carb limit, it is keto friendly. You can also eat an apple a day (depending on the size) but you need to remember the essence of ketosis and take your carbs from energetic sources like protein and healthy fats. Once you are able to understand the difference between non-keto and keto-friendly foods; you will notice that ketosis is not that tough after all.

- **Calculation is Important:**

The best way to transit in ketosis is to keep a track of your carbs. This might seem annoying at first, but gradually, you will see how helpful it is and you will eventually understand the importance of calculating the net carbs per day. It is extremely crucial and usually people overlook this issue quite easily. However, if you want to settle into ketosis perfectly; it is best that you keep a track of your net carbs.

- **Set an Environment:**

Most of the people who struggle at ketosis are the ones who don't set their environment according to it. Remember the section of "stocking up your fridge?" Well, that is the basic step towards settling your environment. You certainly cannot expect your surroundings to be filled with ice cream, candies, chocolates and nuts and hope to settle for a huge dietary lifestyle change, can you? It is somewhat impossible. Thus, the best way to transit into ketosis, is to set your atmosphere accordingly. Clean your pantry, make a list of healthy, low carb foods and go to the grocery store to stock up on them. Bring a limitation to the variety of food that is accessible at your home and plan your meals ahead. Put a meal plan in front of your desk every week, so that you always have an eye on it.

- **Mindful Eating:**

Mindful eating is a very important step towards transition into ketosis. Your caloric intake has a huge impact on your weight loss. The more calories you take, the harder it gets to lose the stubborn, stored fat. A keto calculator can be extremely helpful in this matter though. You can calculate your caloric intake on the go and limit your food intake accordingly. Also, before you pick something to eat, you can instantly calculate the calories you will be take in. This is known as mindful eating; knowing what you are eating and how is it going to affect you.

Ketosis is all about gaining knowledge and getting into the habit of mindful eating. Once you have the knowledge about what you are eating and how much does it has to offer to you; you are gradually going to see major changes taking place in your overall diet routine. You will also find yourself adjusting to ketosis much easier.

Part 2-Step by Step Guide To Intermittent Fasting

Chapter 4: What Is Intermittent Fasting?

Intermittent fasting is a pattern of dieting as you skip meals consciously. This is one of the most used methods or type of ketosis.

In intermittent fasting, one fasts for around 12-36 hours, skipping meals purposely. It is reported to be one of the best ways to manage weight amazingly. There are many perks of intermittent fasting, like enhanced brain functions, weight loss and reduction in chronic illnesses too.

Intermittent fasting has two basic types:

- 16/8 hour window
- 24 hour window

In order to understand them in depth, here is a detailed summary of these two types of fasting.

- **16/8 hour Fasting:**

In this type of intermittent fasting, you fast for around 16 hours and then eat your carbs and healthy fats and proteins, within the next 8 hour window. This definitely means that you will be skipping your breakfast. You can either skip breakfast or dinner, depending on the time that is easier to fast. Usually it is best that you do not eat anything from 8pm onwards and skip breakfast. Many people also eat during a 4 hour window. This is termed as feasting as your body produces ketones much rapidly in it. This 16/8 hour style intermittent fasting is the most preferred style of fasting and is also very helpful in weight management.

For example, if you start eating at 2pm then you need to stop eating at 10pm till 16 hours. Likewise, if you start eating at 7am, you need to stop eating at 3pm and fast for the next 16 hours. However, you also need to make sure that you do not stick to fasting for more than 3 days per week.

- **24 Hour Fasting:**

The other type of intermittent fasting is the 24 hour one. You eat your last meal at 8pm and then you do not eat anything till the next day, 8pm. This obviously means that you will be skipping all three meals of the day. Also, it is not important top push yourself till 8pm. it really depends on your stamina too and it is best if you don't cross your limitations a lot. If you are able to perform a 20 hour or an

18 hour fast too; it is good. Just make sure that a 24 hour fast crosses the 16 hour lapse.

These are the basic two types of intermittent fasting, where 16/8 hour fasting is the most preferred one till yet. It is considered the most effective way to lose and manage weight. Furthermore, your body stays in the phase of ketosis in a much enhanced manner through intermittent fasting. Also, fasting does not mean that you can eat aimlessly and meaninglessly, all the time. Knowing when to stop and what to eat is very important.

The Science behind Intermittent Fasting;

The first thought that strikes the human mind is that skipping a meal or two or all the meals for an entire day, is obviously going to help you in losing weight. With low caloric intake, you obviously allow your body to lose more weight and much rapidly as well.

According to science, fasting every other day is equivalent to eating less and in control, each day. However, the basic problem with a constant healthy lifestyle is that it gets tiring for the dieter. Some days, you just don't feel like controlling and eating in a balance. Thus, the science behind intermittent fasting is to make it better and easier for everyone.

Maintaining a healthy weight is hard. Once you stop controlling over your eating portions, it will take just a few weeks and your weight loss efforts will turn to ash. With intermittent fasting, you are able to simplify things largely. It is more like a hack for people who want to maintain a good weight and in a simpler manner, without the hassle of meal planning or cooking on their own.

Benefits of Intermittent Fasting

Looking beyond the perks of weight loss, there is a lot more that intermittent fasting has to offer. According to studies, this diet style has a lot of health benefits and is extremely powerful too. In order to understand the goodness of this type of ketosis, we have summed up the basic perks of intermittent fasting below:

- **Weight Loss:**
  The basic advantage that intermittent fasting has to offer is weight loss. It is the core reason why people tend to rely on this style of ketosis. The science behind intermittent fasting is to eat less and take few calories. Fasting enhances your metabolism system which helps massively in burning calories. Thus, through reduction of food intake and increased metabolism, the stored fat is accessed and burnt, while you are fasting. This boosts the weight loss and helps you in losing your belly fat too.

- **Reduces Oxidative Stress:**

    Oxidative stress is the core reason behind several chronic illnesses. It also boosts anti-aging signs and makes you feel dimmer and older way before time. Different studies show that intermittent fasting helps in reduction of oxidative stress and enhances inflammation too.

- **Stronger Heart:**

    According to science, cardiovascular diseases are one of the major causes of deaths, throughout the world. An unhealthy heart, cannot survive for long, can it? Unhealthy eating is the major cause of cardiovascular diseases. Intermittent fasting can actually make your heart health amazing as it balances the blood pressure, blood sugar levels and cholesterol levels too.

- **Happier and Healthier Brain:**

    Intermittent fasting helps in reducing oxidative stress which eventually puts your brain in a state of peace. Through this style of ketosis, various aspects of human metabolism are improved which boost the brain health too. A stable metabolic system is able to reduce excessive inflammation, balance the blood sugar levels and also bring in insulin resistance. All of this, not only enhances your brain's ability to think and act, but it also tends to boost its creativity and reduce issues like anxiety and depression.

Through intermittent fasting, you are not just losing weight or your stubborn belly fat. You are able to attain a lot more than just weight loss. You are boosting your internal system and are striving to be healthier from within. A healthy heart and a creative and productive brain are the two basic entities which make you capable of spending a healthy lifestyle.

Autophagy:

Autophagy is an unfamiliar term to many but people, who opt for intermittent fasting, usually do have knowledge about it. This is a process through which the human body is able to clean out the unneeded and old cellular material from the body. It also removes any of the unwanted material that might cause damage or any diseases. However, the human body only enters the state of autophagy through fasting.

Now, the studies that have proven autophagy to be an important phase of ketosis; it is essential to remember that these researches have been done on mice. Tests are hard to be done on humans, relating this process; however, it is not impossible. It is said that the human body enters the stage of autophagy, after 18-20 hours of fasting. Therefore, if you fast for an entire day, your body has already entered autophagy and has probably removed a lot of waste material from it. Therefore, autophagy is the basic element that makes the 24 hour intermittent fasting incredible. Attaining autophagy requires a serious commitment towards a 24 hour fast and if you wish to attain it; there is literally no other way to do so.

How Fasting burns Fat?

As the major perk of intermittent fasting is weight loss; it is important to understand that how does fasting actually burns the stored fat. In this brief outline, we will be describing how one can burn fat, through fasting.

Firstly, fasting is not a new invention at all. It has been practiced religiously, since years by the Muslim, Christian and Monk community. It has been centuries since the term of fasting has surfaced and even though there are several myths that state fasting has life endangering; nothing negative has ever happened to people who practice it.

Now, as the core focus of intermittent fasting is weight loss; how does your body burn fat while fasting? Through fasting, your body is left with only one choice; to tap into the stored fat, looking for energy, to go throughout the day, without taking anything further. The human body works on two basic fuels; sugar and fat and you cannot burn both of them, at the same time, right? You either have to burn sugar or you can burn fat.

Usually the body tends to burn sugar faster because it is easier, in comparison to burning fats. Thus, the human body burns sugar first and by the time it moves towards burning fats; you are up for your next meal. This leads to hormonal imbalance and weight gain and water retention too. This does sound familiar, doesn't it? Don't worry as it happens to everyone. However, fasting is a much simplified manner which helps you in escaping this never ending cycle and actually loses weight.

When you fast, your body is restricted from all types of calories. With no intake of food, your body starts using up the sugar as the only source of energy. Fasting for 16 or 20 hours is a long time span and even if you think that it isn't; it is actually helping you in several ways. As sugar burns faster, your body will eventually switch up to the fat store and will start burning fat. Also, once the sugar has been used, your body will have low glycogen level which will make your kidneys get rid of excessive water too. Thus, you won't only be losing weight but will also be able to fight issues like water retention and hormonal imbalance etc. so, it is a win-win situation, as you will be losing weight, burning your stored fats and will also be providing your body with other healthy perks.

Everything runs on Hormones:

Hormones are the most important messengers of human body and this is why, an imbalance in them, can create havoc within. They are responsible for sending the signals from the body to the brain and vice versa. As they are the crucial agents of adaption and protection, they have the ability to hinder the brain performance as well. For instance, a boost in stress hormones can alter brain functioning and the abilities of the brain to learn and adapt to new things. Similarly, sexual hormones are responsible for sending in signals to the brain, to feel emotions and sensual. A lot of people, who complain that they don't feel the sexual drive, are usually reported to have a great imbalance in their hormones. Likewise, many people who are unable to lose weight, despite their endless efforts, usually come to acknowledge the fact that they have excessive hormonal issues which are not making them lose their fat. Thus, we need to understand that everything runs on hormones. Your body is actually running in hormone production and if they are not in a good equilibrium or near to a good and balanced state; it has the ability to mess up with the entire human system easily. This brief outline is going to be carried out in the next chapter which will portray how intermittent fasting helps you in achieving a good hormonal balance and keeping your body healthy.

Chapter 5: Hormones VS Fasting; How does it work?

The perks of intermittent fasting are literally abuzz in the world of healthy living. It has tons of advantages, apart from just weight loss which is why, it has gathered immense appreciation. In the light of several studies, intermittent fasting helps in enhancing the metabolism system, boosts cellular repair and also heals an unhealthy gut. Therefore, there is no visible reason to not praise intermittent fasting.

Restricting food intake can actually help you in losing weight and is definitely beneficial in several other ways. But it can be a little messy for your hormones, if you do not attend to it properly.

First of all, fasting has a great connection with the most important hormones, progesterone and estrogen. The brain releases hormones to the ovaries to release progesterone and estrogen. If this axis, through which the signals are sent to the ovaries, is not in great health shape, it can cause several health issues, for both men and women.

Now, women are extremely sensitive in this manner and if intermittent fasting is not done right, it can actually lead to infertility issues as well. This is where, a balance has to be obtained so that fasting can boost the hormonal performance and not cause an issue for it. It is important that a cycle should be set up for fasting. You don't need to fast consecutively for 4-5 days. Two days per week is just fine and make sure that you don't set consecutive days for fasting. For women, it is best to fast maximum for 16 hours and not does any intense workouts during fasting. Light running or brisk walk is perfect. If you are able to feel that your body is getting stronger and your stamina is not dropping by every time you fast; then it is safe to go for. You must understand how intermittent fasting works to benefit from it. Don't overdo your fasts and don't push your limits to an extent where you feel dizzy all the time.

This being said, intermittent fasting can actually bring you a balance in hormones too. Yet again, you need to attend to this plan properly, to avail the benefits.

When you fast, making sure that you balance your nutrients during the time when you are not fasting, you are able to bring a balance between cortisol and melatonin. This is the key factor which a lot of people don't pay much attention to while attending to intermittent fasting. When you opt for this style of ketosis, you actually bring a great stability between these two hormones which is able to provide you with great energy levels and a wonderful sleeping pattern too.

Secondly, intermittent fasting can also enhance hormone growth. If your hormones are not growing with time, it means that you will soon run out of the balance. This is where fasting really helps as it boosts hormone growth and helps in muscle growth and repair too.

Thus, the basic advice to take away from this piece of information is that fasting is definitely a very amazing manner to lose weight and boost your health too. However, if it is not done correctly, under the provided guidelines, it can create havoc for the hormones. As hormones run the human body, they must not be neglected at all. Therefore, make sure that while you are not fasting; you are providing your body with good and healthy nutrients so that it can run efficiently while fasting.

Role of Insulin in Human Body:

The responsibility of insulin is to regulate the blood sugar levels and keep glucose balanced. If the body lacks insulin heavily, it puts an individual to risk of diabetes. Insulin plays a very important role for the metabolic system as it regulates how glucose and fat is used and stored in the body. Several body cells rely on insulin for performing adequately.

Insulin and Intermittent Fasting:

Now that you know the role of insulin in human body, it is time to see how intermittent fasting benefits the control of this hormone. According to studies, fasting can actually be advantageous for enhancing blood sugar levels. This is extremely helpful for people who might be at risk of diabetes. Also, both types of intermittent fasting (the ones stated above) are equally beneficial for reducing the insulin resistance and controlling the blood sugar levels. Furthermore, when the blood sugar levels are in control, the risk of sudden rise in sugar levels is heavily reduced. However, fasting has different effects on men and women and a little variation can occur in the balancing of blood sugar levels, on gender basis.

Meet your Hunger Hormones; Leptin and Ghrelin:

Leptin and Ghrelin are the two basic hunger hormones of the human body. So if you feel hungry quite often, you must know that these two are definitely not in balance. Leptin is created through fat cells and is responsible for decreasing your appetite. On the contrary, Ghrelin is a hormone which increases your appetite. Thus, if they both are not stable; you are either going to feel extremely hungry almost all the time or you won't feel the hunger mostly. Also, Ghrelin is the hormones which play a vital role in weight loss and management.

To begin with, Ghrelin is an appetite booster and is found in the stomach which sends hunger signals to the human brain. Ghrelin increases if an individual is under eating and vice versa. According to science, ghrelin plays a crucial role in determining the hunger levels and how often it kicks back in the stomach. Ghrelin obviously spikes up before you eat as it symbolizes hunger. As soon as you eat, ghrelin level is lowered for almost the next 3 hours.

Secondly, Leptin plays a huge role in the human body and it is safe to say, that is more vital than ghrelin. This is because it determines the energy levels of a person, even though it is an appetite suppressor. Leptin signals the brain to suppress hunger and timeless cravings and pushes the body to use the stored fat, as a source of energy. However, obese people are usually unable to react to Leptin, which leads them to overate and boost ghrelin levels. Studies show that Leptin is high in people who are fat but they are unable to respond to it as ghrelin is always making them feel hungry.

How are both these diets a miracle for burning fat?

The ketosis bandwagon is huge and with every passing day, several people are jumping towards it, to attain the benefits that it has to offer. They not only accelerate your weight loss but also boost several other health benefits too. Ketosis and intermittent fasting have the ability to turn your body into a fat burning machine and also enhance your brain's abilities.

As both of these diets focus on low caloric intake and aim at providing healthy fats and proteins to the body; they are able to enhance the overall health of an individual. When you fast for 16 hours and eat in an 8 hour window, following the ketosis nutritional facts, you are able to lose a lot more fat than usual. As ketosis emphasizes upon low carb intake and moderate protein intake, along with healthy fats; your body gets everything that it needs, in order to run efficiently. If you eat junk while following the intermittent fasting, it won't bring a huge difference in your overall weight at all. It is important that you eat healthy while you are on ketogenic diet or intermittent fasting. This is the major reason why a lot of people tend to combine intermittent fasting with keto diet. Through the combination, people are able to burn more fat and manage their weight wonderfully well. According to studies, people who keep their carb intake low while intermittent fasting are able to lose 10-20% fatter in comparison to people who rely on junk food and unhealthy eating items after fasting for 16 hours. The 8 hour window that you are provided with needs to be availed smartly. Load up with protein and healthy fats and some berries so that your body gets the elements that are easier and faster to burn.

The 21 Day Meal Plans:

Switching to ketogenic diet plan can be a little difficult but it really depends upon you, as to how you want to deal with it. The basic rule is that the lower the carb intake, the faster you enter the state of ketosis. Thus, sticking to keto friendly foods is going to be the key to gain success in keto diet.

In this chapter, we will be providing you with a 21 day meal plan which will help you in reaching ketosis and attaining the benefits of it, at its best. You will realize that ketosis is not that tough but dieters actually make it difficult for themselves. With these scrumptious meals, you can actually have the best keto diet and lose weight, without feeling sympathetic for yourself. Eating healthy is certainly the key.

Week 1:

Day 1:

Monday

- **Breakfast; Scrambled Eggs:**

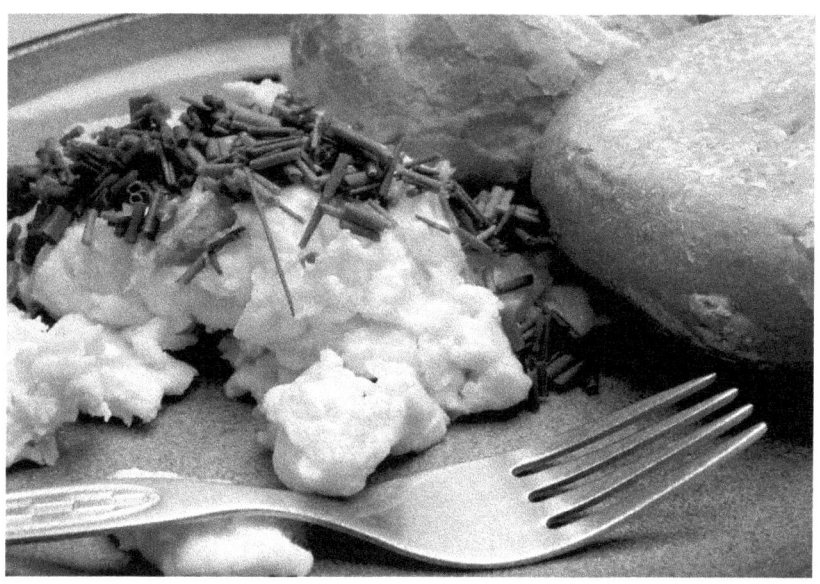

Eggs and butter are the best combination for a perfect, keto friendly breakfast. Starting your day off with it is going to bring the most satisfying and energetic breakfast to your table.

Ingredients:

You will need;

- Butter-1 oz.
- Egss-2
- Salt and Pepper- accordig to taste

Preparation:

Crack and whisk the eggs in a bowl and add salt and pepper to it. Melt the butter on low-medium heat and make sure that it does not burn. Once the butter has melted, pour the eggs in the pan and stir it for a minute or two, until it is cooked and creamy. Have a healthy and satisfying breakfast!

- **Lunch: Keto No Noodle Chicken Soup:**

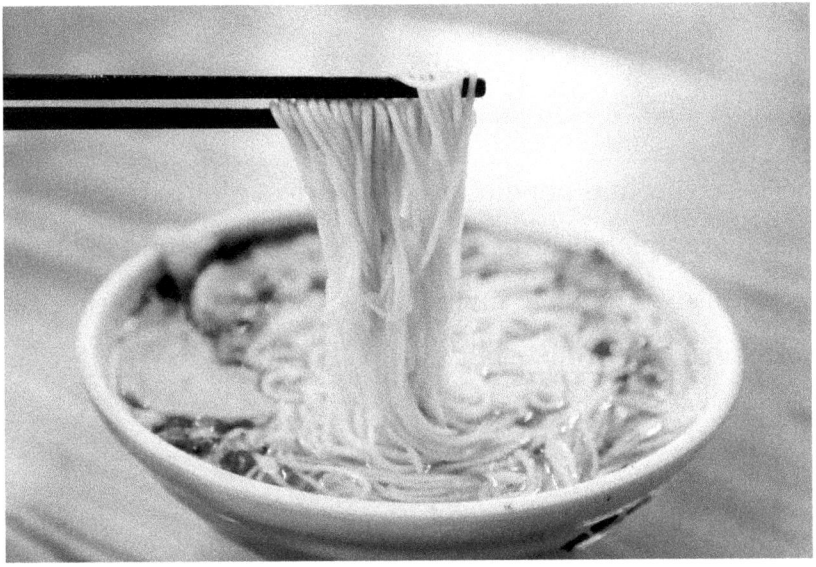

This is a healthy and comforting noodle chicken soup, which is made out of healing bone broth and also helps you in fighting a stubborn cold or flu. Filled with nutrition, this is the best keto friendly lunch to have on a cold day.

- **Dinner: Keto Carbonara:**

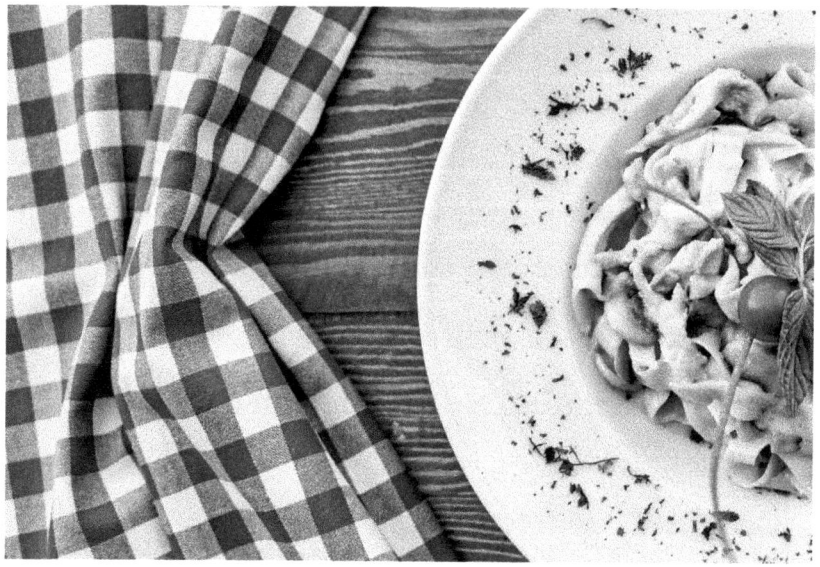

These zucchini noodles are the perfect alternative to pasta and are much healthier. The creamy texture and the crispy bacon are enough to make you feel the mouthwatering dish, kicking in your taste buds.

Day 2:
Tuesday:

- **Breakfast: Keto Frittata with Fresh Spinach:**

Eye catching and easy to make, this is an impressive and yummy breakfast for keto dieters. The magical combo of spinach, bacon, sausage and eggs is perfect for the right kick of energy needed early in the morning.

- **Lunch; Keto Asian Beef Salad:**

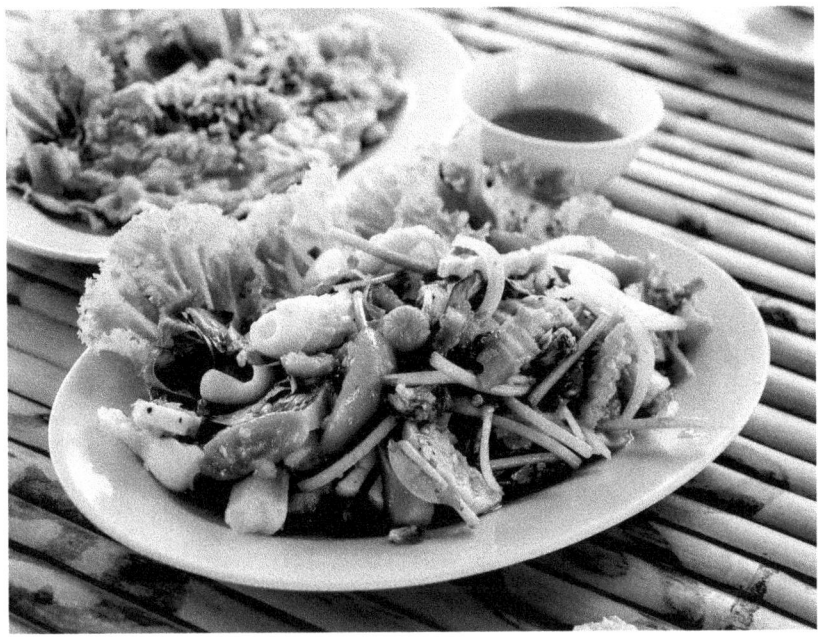

The perfect savory taste with a gingery kick is all you need to boost your mood and taste buds in the noon, with a fulfilling meal.

Ingredients:

You will need;

- For the Beef:
- Olive Oil-1 tbsp.
- Fish Sauce-1 tbsp.
- Chili Flakes- 1 tsp.
- Grated fresh ginger-1 tbsp.
- Rib eye Steaks-2/3 lb.
- For Sesame Mayonnaise:
- Dijon Mustard-1 tsp.
- Egg Yolk-1

- Avocado Oil-1/2 cup
- Sesame Oil-1 tbsp.
- Lime Juice-1/2 tbsp.
- Salt and Pepper
- Salad:
- Scallions-2
- Cherry Tomatoes- 3 oz.
- Cucumber- 2 oz.
- Red onion-1/2
- Sesame seeds-1 tbsp.
- Fresh Cilantro

Preparation:

Start with making the sesame mayonnaise, by mixing the Dijon mustard and egg yolk together. Whisk continuously and gradually keep adding the avocado oil. Don't add it all at once; slow and steady is the trick. A hand mixer will be great in this. Once done, add the lime juice, sesame oil and salt and pepper and give it a final mix. Make sure that the mayonnaise is emulsified.

Now, combine all the ingredients of the beef in a plastic bag and add the beef to it. Marinade it for 15 minutes, at room temperature. Put it aside and chop all the veggies for the salad, in bite size pieces, leaving the scallions behind. Divide the vegetables into two sections.

Now, toast the sesame seeds on medium heat until they are light brown. Set them aside. Now, pat the beef dry with the help of a paper towel and fry it on high heat, for a minute or two, on both sides. Make sure that it is cooked to medium. Once done, fry scallions in this same pan and then slice the meat into thin slices. Now, place the vegetables in a bowl and top it with beef slices, scallions. Serve along with sesame mayonnaise and roasted seeds.

- **Dinner: Baked Salmon with Asparagus:**

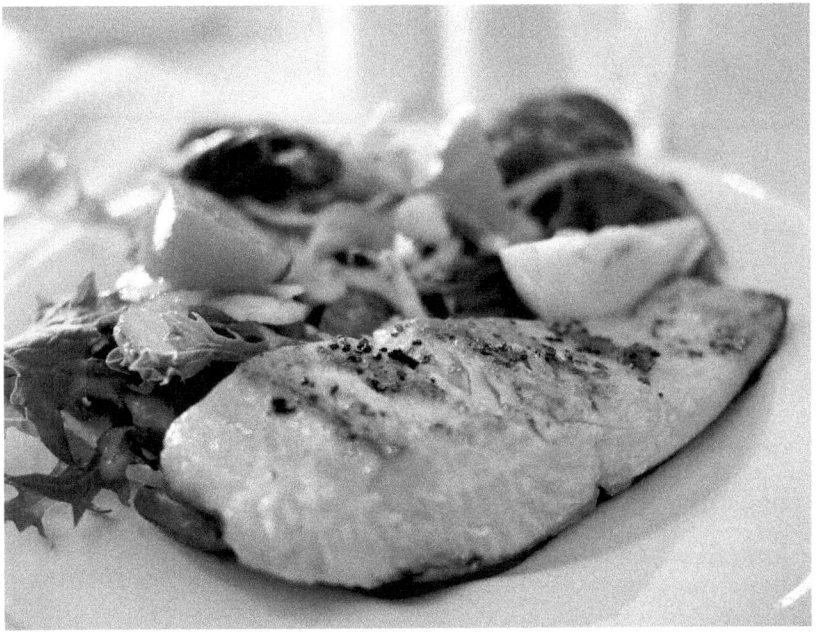

This is a beautiful dish which is made with a heavenly combination of a simple sauce made of lemon juice, butter salt and pepper. Make your taste buds feel amazing before the end of the day!

DAY 3:

Wednesday:

- **Breakfast: 3 Egg Omelet with Spinach, Sausage and Cheese**

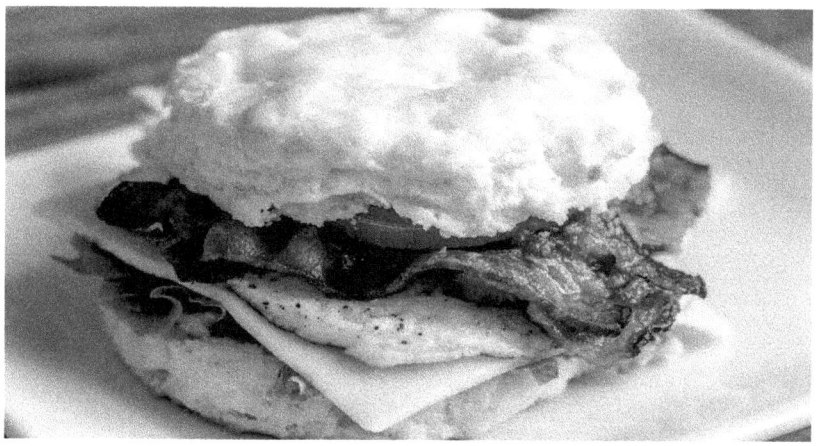

Eggs are packed with protein and are the best way to start off the day. This is an extremely healthy omelet to kick your day off and have the right levels of energy too while on ketosis.

- **BLT Salad:**

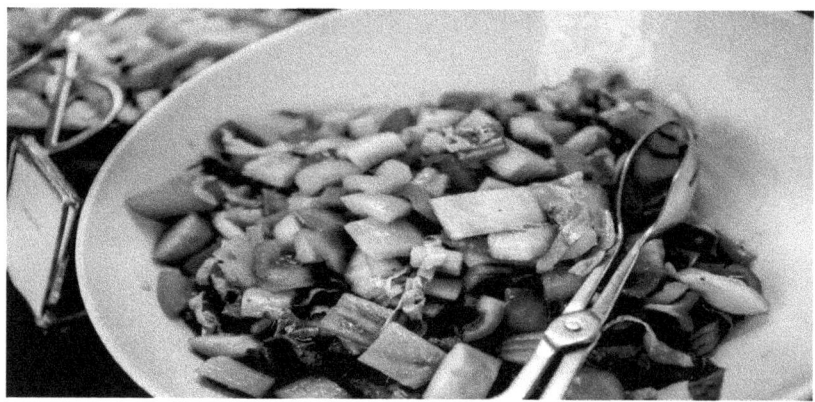

A combination of lettuce, tomato and bacon is all you need to make this keto friendly salad for your lunch!

- **Dinner; Keto Pesto Casserole:**

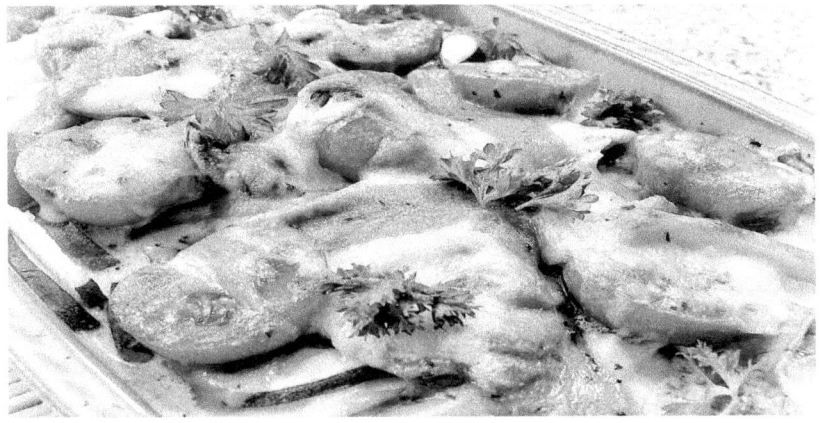

This is a very easy to make keto dish which is creamy and delicious to its core. Have the most scrumptious and low carb dinner!

Ingredients:

You will need:

- Boneless Chicken Breast-1 ½ lbs.
- Coconut Oil or Butter-2 tbsp.
- Pitted Olives-3 oz.
- Diced Feta Cheese-5 oz.

- Salt and Pepper
- Heavy whipping cream-1 ¼ cups
- Green Pesto or red pesto-3 oz.
- Finely chopped garlic clove-1
- For Serving:
- Olive Oil-4 tbsp.

- Leafy Greens-5 oz.
- Ground black pepper
- Sea Salt

Preparation:

Preheat the oven to 200 C and cut the chicken breast into bite sized pieces. Season it with salt and pepper. Take a large skillet and add butter to it. Sautee the chicken pieces in it on medium flame until they are golden brown.

Now, mix together pesto and heavy cream in a bowl.

Take a baking dish and put the sautéed chicken pieces along with feta cheese and garlic and pesto. Bake them for 20-30 minutes. The dish should be a little golden and bubbly from the edges which showcases that it is done and ready to be eaten.

Day 4:
Thursday:

- **Breakfast: Keto Cheese Roll Ups:**

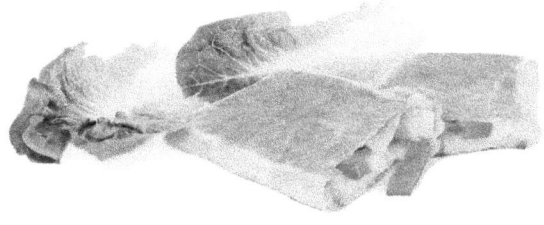

The simplest and yummiest breakfast to make is the keto cheese rolls up which are packed with savory goodness perfectly.

Ingredients:

You will need:

- Cheddar cheese- 8 oz.
- Butter-2 oz.

Preparations:

Put the cheese slices on a cutting board and cut butter into very thin slices with the help of a knife or a cheese slicer. Cover each cheese slice with the thin slice of butter and roll it up. THAT IS IT. The easiest and quickest breakfast to make which is very healthy and keto friendly.

- **Lunch: Keto Caprese Omelet:**

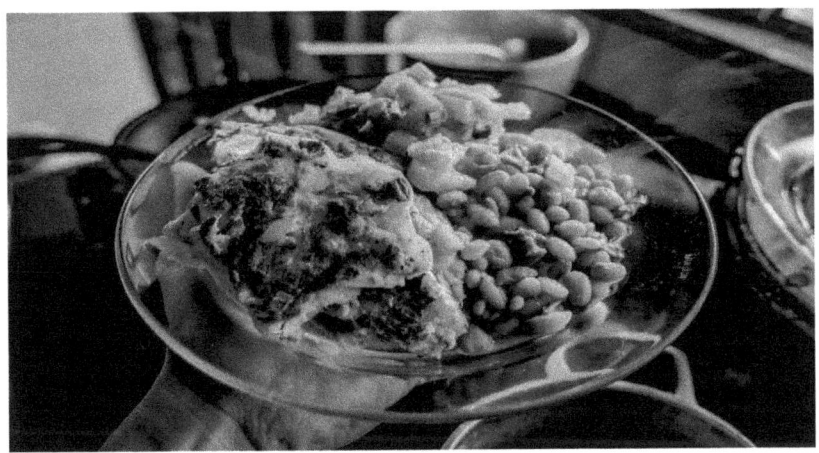

This keto friendly dish can be used for lunch, breakfast or dinner as it is very easy and quick to make and tastes heavenly too. It has the perfect Italy tastes and is nothing less than scrumptious.

- **Dinner: Keto Meat Pie**

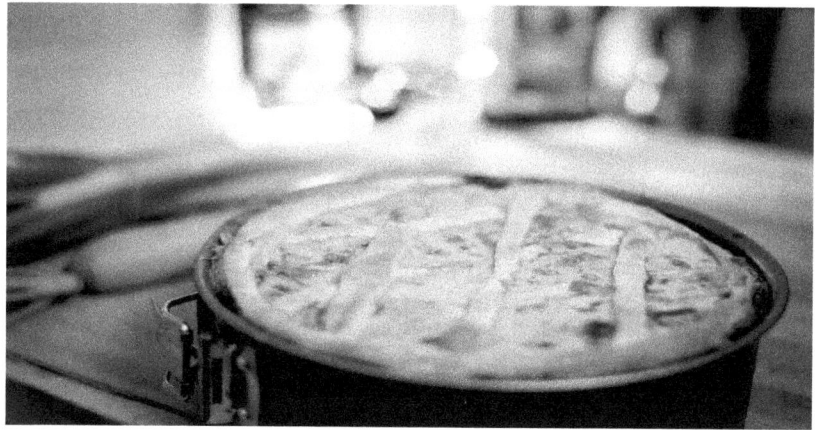

Topped with cheese, this is an incredible keto meat pie which is wonderfully satisfying. Serving it warm is going to burst out flavors like none other.

Day 5:
Friday

- **Breakfast: Dairy Free Keto Latte:**

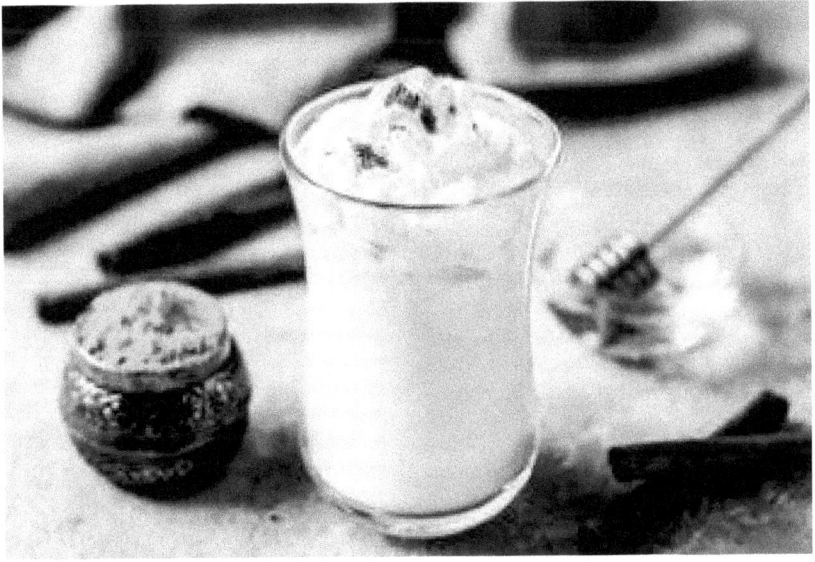

Latte lovers, this is the best pick for you for breakfast if you are on keto diet. Within just 5 minutes, you can have your dairy free keto latte ready to soothe your taste buds which have probably missed latte badly.

- **Lunch: Keto Avocado, Bacon and Goat Cheese Salad:**

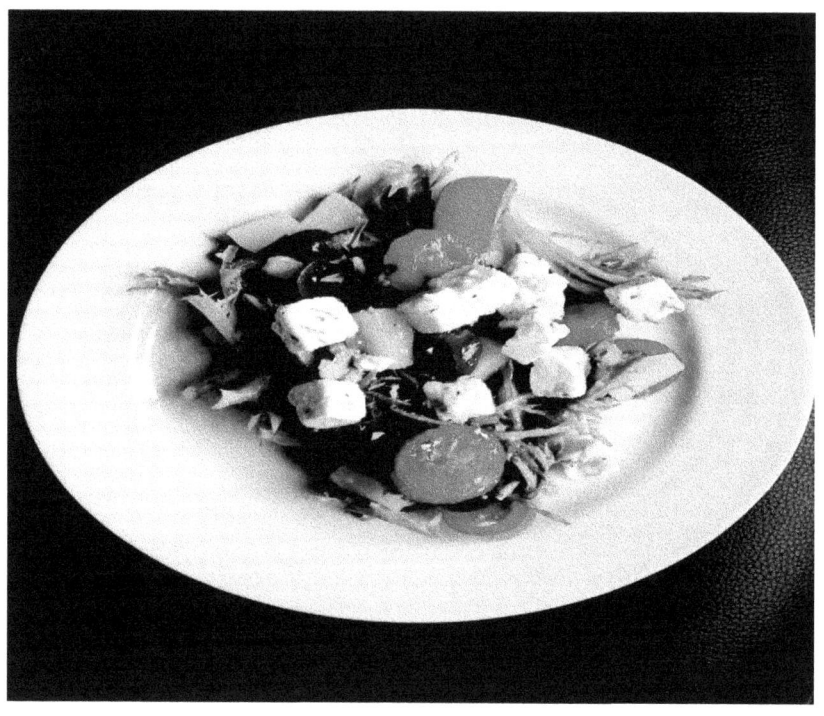

This is the boss keto salad which keeps your lunch quite light and tasty.

Ingredients:

- You will need:
- Lemon Juice-1/2
- Olive Oil-1/2 cup
- Mayonnaise-1/2 cup

Preparation:

Spread parchment paper on a baking dish and preheat your own on 200 degree Celsius.

Cut the goat cheese into 1cm rounds slices and place them on the parchment paper. Back them until they are golden.

Until the cheese is being baked, fry the bacon until they are crispy. Now, cut avocado in your desired size pieces and place them on the arugula. Top it with the crispy fried bacon and goat cheese and finish it by sprinkling some nuts on it.

For the dressing, blend lemon juice, olive oil and mayonnaise with an immersion blender. If you want, you can add a tablespoon or two of whipping cream to it too. Season it with salt and pepper and serve right away.

- **Dinner: Keto Pizza:**

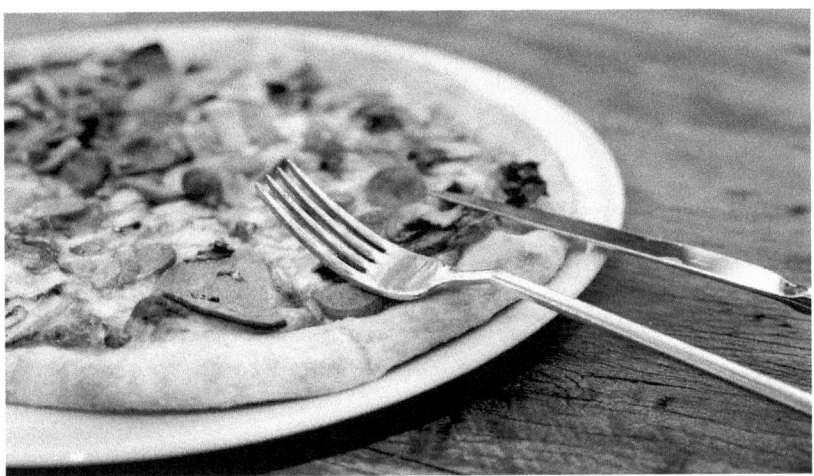

Who doesn't love pizza? We all do and if you are ketosis and you have a heavy craving for the best pizza, then you can rely on the keto pizza for sure. With lesser carbs, you can get your fix for the pizza craving and get the best taste too.

Day 6:
Friday:

- **Breakfast: Mushroom Omelet:**

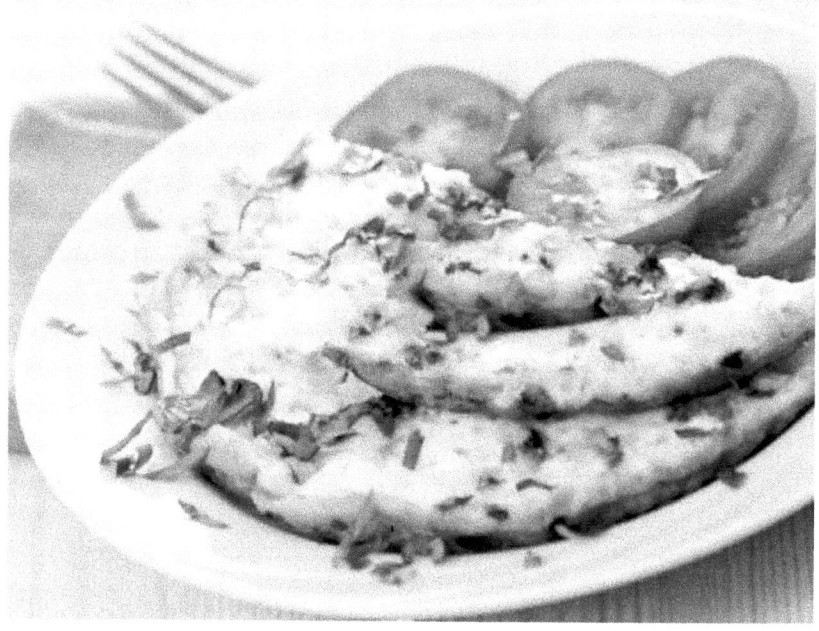

This is an extremely healthy omelet; just take a few minutes to be made. With the mouthwatering filling of mushrooms, nothing beats this omelet as you are able to start your day off wonderfully.

- **Lunch: Keto Smoked Salmon:**

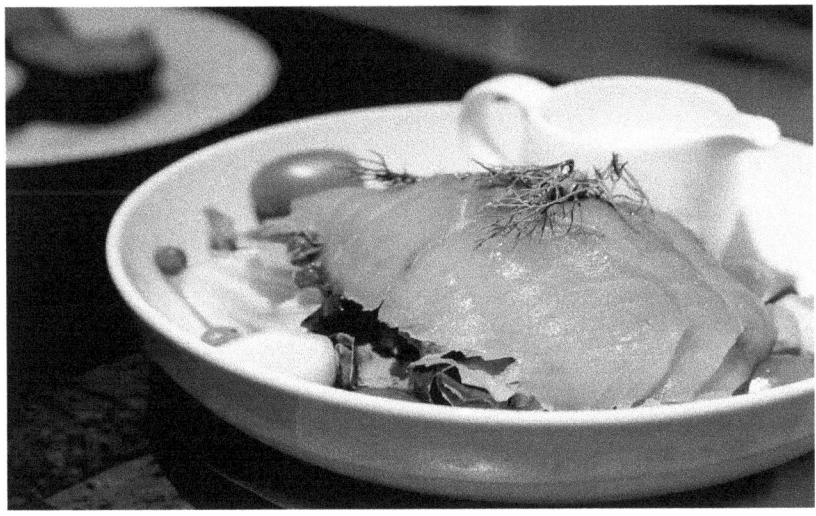

Keto smoked salmon is a real dish on plate which has all the basic needs of the human body. Spinach, lime, salmon and mayo; you get your carbs, protein and healthy fats all in one plate with this amazing lunch meal.

- **Dinner: Keto Asian Cabbage Stir Fry:**

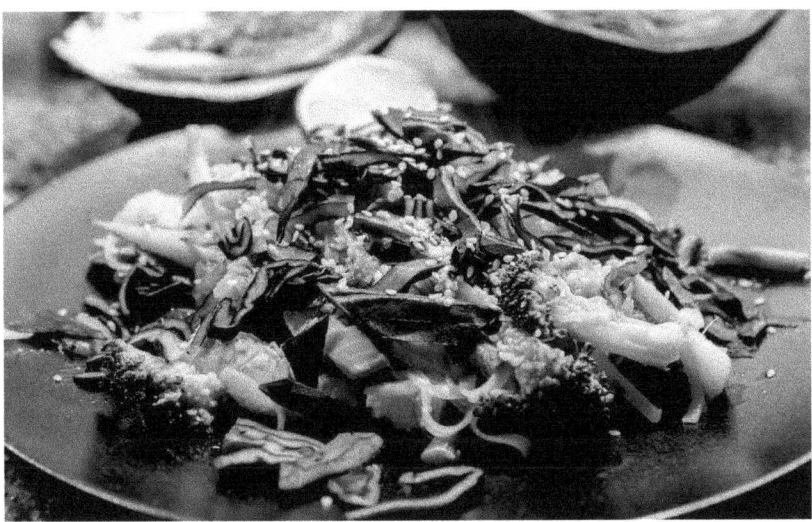

This stir fry brings various colors to your dish, making it appealing in look and taste both. It is crunchy and has a punch of wonderful flavors to it, which is perfect for a dinner meal.

Ingredients:

- You will need:
- Green cabbage-1 ½ lbs.
- Butter; divided- 4oz.
- Salt-1 tsp.
- Onion powder-1 tsp.
- Ground black pepper-¼ tsp.
- White wine vinegar-1 tbsp.
- Minced garlic cloves- 2
- Chili flakes- 1 tsp.
- Finely chopped fresh ginger- 1 tbsp.
- Ground beef- 1 ¼ lbs.
- Chopped scallions- 3 (1/2 inch slices)
- Sesame oil- 1 tbsp.

Preparation:

With the help of a sharp knife, shred the cabbage and fry it, in half of the butter (half of the amount mentioned in the ingredients). Allow the cabbage to turn soft (it can take a little while). Add the mentioned spices and vinegar to the cabbage, once it softens. Stir it for a minute or two so that the spices are mixed together properly. Once done, take the cabbage out in a separate bowl and melt the remaining butter in the same pan. Add garlic, ginger and chili flakes to the butter and sauté them for a while.

Now add the ground meat to it and let it cook until the meat has been cooked perfectly and the juices have evaporated. Once the meat is cooked, lower down the flame and adds the cabbage and scallions to it. Stir until everything is combined and season it with salt and pepper. Dish it out and sprinkle sesame seeds on it.

To make the wasabi mayonnaise, mix a little amount of wasabi paste in the mayonnaise, and then keep stirring it until combined. Add the wasabi according to your taste and serve it along the cabbage stir fry.

Day 7:
Sunday:

- **Breakfast: Keto Pancakes with Whipped Cream and Berries:**

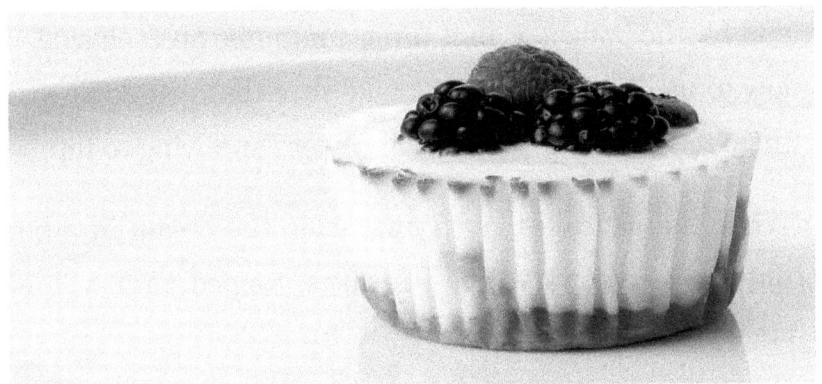

Starting your Sunday with these pancakes is the best idea for a wonderfully satisfied and delicious breakfast. These amazing cottage cheese pancakes will make you forget the old school ones!

Ingredients:

You will need:

- Eggs-4
- Cottage Cheese-4 oz.
- Coconut Oil-2 oz.
- Ground psyllium husk powder-1 tbsp.
- <u>For the topping, you will need:</u>
- Raspberries-1/2 cup
- Heavy whipping cream-1 cup

Preparation:

Mix together the eggs, psyllium husk powder and cottage cheese and set it aside for around 15 minutes so that it thickens a bit. Take a non-stick skillet and heat butter in it and fry the pancakes in it for 3-4 minutes on each side, on low to medium heat. Also, make sure that you don't make them too big because they will be very annoying to flip.

While the pancakes are frying, whip the cream in a bowl until it is soft. Serve the pancakes, topped with whipped cream and berries.

- **Lunch: Italian Keto Plate:**

If you want your Sunday to be a bit lazy and stress free, then this is the perfect meal for you. It is very easy to put together and has all the basics that will energize your mood and body!

- **Dinner: Keto Tortilla with Ground Beef and Salsa:**

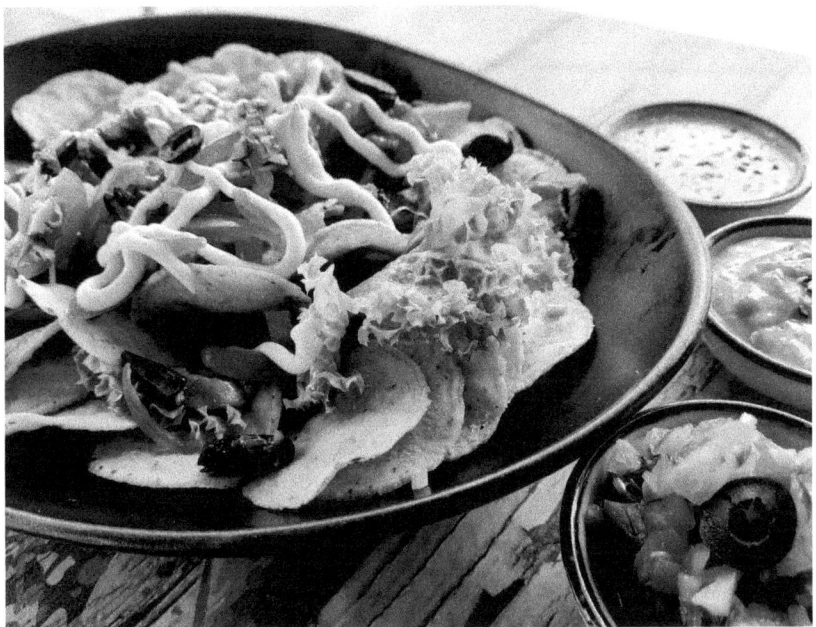

A tortilla wrapped with meat and cheese is nothing less than a treat in dinner, right? With your own homemade, keto style bread, this tortilla is going to quench the thirst of your taste buds really well.

Week 2:
Day 8:
Monday:

- **Breakfast: No bread, keto breakfast sandwich:**

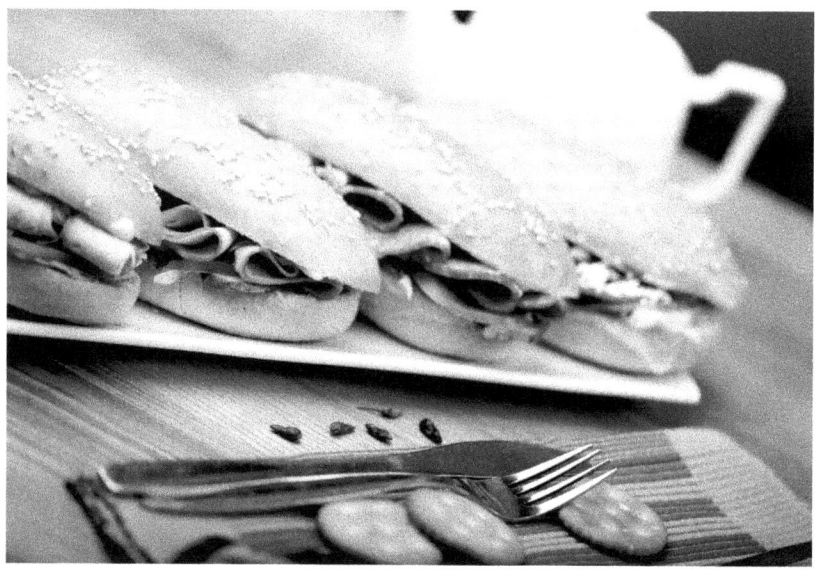

The perfect combo of ham and eggs with a punch of cheese, makes the best ever breakfast sandwich that you would want for yourself to beat down the Monday blues.

- **Lunch: Keto Tuna Salad with Boiled Eggs:**

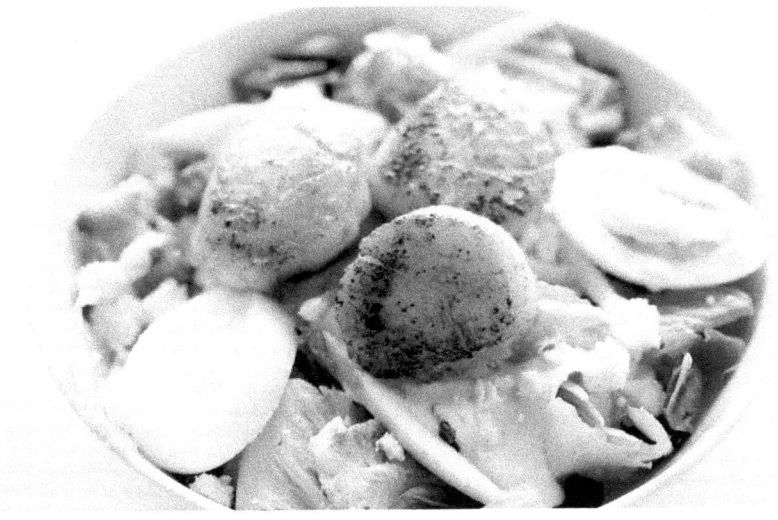

Don't have time to fix a huge meal for your lunch on a busy Monday? Well, this just needs 15 minutes and is one of the best lunch meals that you would ever want. With all the healthy and wholesome ingredients, this is the perfect "oh-so keto" dish!

Ingredients:

You will need:

- Scallions- 2
- Celery stalks-4 oz.
- Mayonnaise- ¾ cup
- Lemon juice and zest- ½
- Dijon Mustard-1 tbsp.
- Tuna in Olive oil-5 oz.
- Cherry tomatoes-4 oz.
- Olive Oil-2 tbsp.
- Salt and pepper

Preparation:

Finely chop the scallions and celery and mix it together with tuna, lemon, mustard and mayonnaise. Stir perfectly so all the ingredients are combined nicely and season it with salt and pepper; put aside.

Boil the eggs and peel them when they are warm. Divide them into half or wedges; as you like them.

Place a romaine lettuce on the plate and spoon out the tuna and eggs on the lettuce. Add tomatoes to the dish and drizzle a bit of olive oil on it. Season a bit with salt and pepper and your lunch is all set!

- **Dinner: Keto Hamburger Patties with Tomato Sauce:**

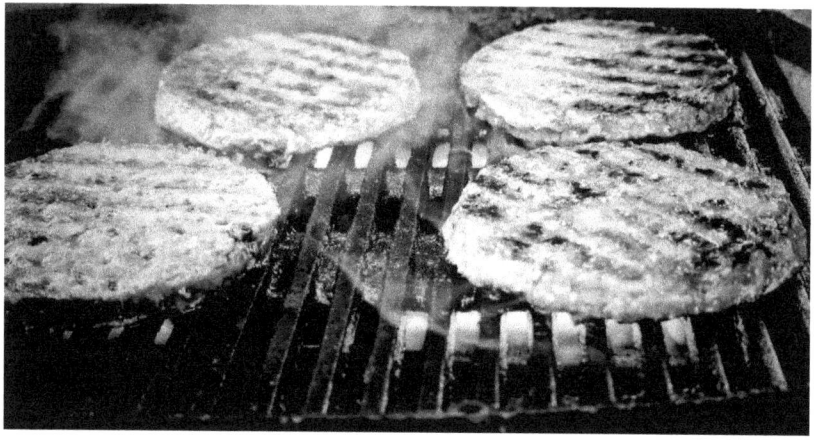

This bun free burger is extremely delicious and the creamy tomato sauce makes it all the more satisfying.

Day 9:
Tuesday:

- **Breakfast: Bulletproof Coffee:**

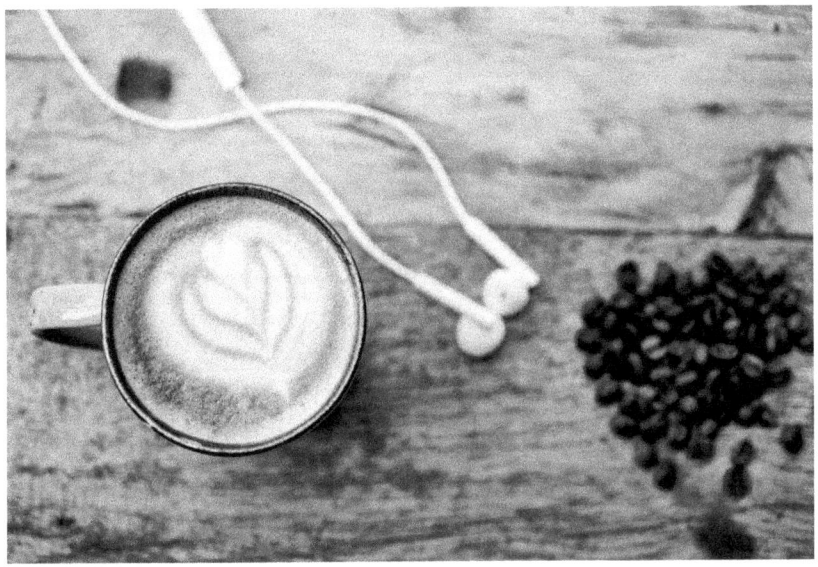

Just a few sips of this coffee and you will literally feel the energy of a bullet taking over you. You can easily take on the world with just this coffee in your breakfast.

- **Lunch: Keto roast beef and cheddar plate:**

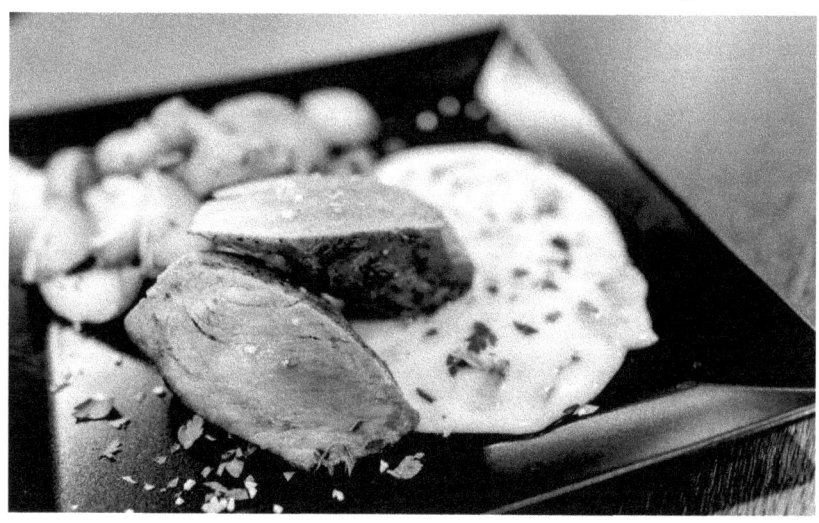

Roasted beef with cheese, scallions, avocados and radishes; this is the perfect real lunch meal for all the keto dieters. And not to forget; it tastes heavenly too.

- **Dinner: Keto Fried Salmon with Broccoli and Cheese:**

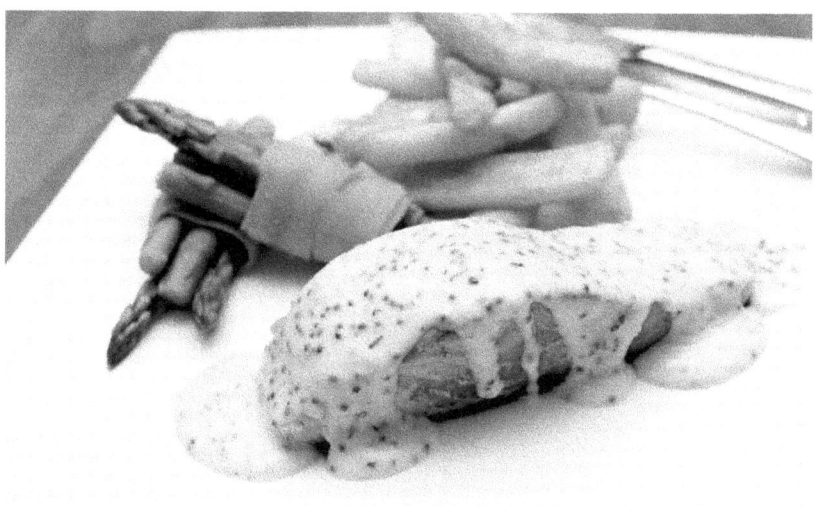

Just in half an hour, this healthy and tasty dish is all done and ready! Here is how to make it:

Ingredients:

You will need:

- Broccoli- 1 lb.
- Butter-3 oz.
- Salt and pepper
- Salmon-1 ½ lbs.
- Grated cheddar cheese-5 oz.
- Lime-1 (optional)

Preparation:

Using the broiler settings of your oven (preferred), preheat your oven at 200 degree Celsius.

Cut the broccoli in small pieces and allow it to drench for a while in salted water for a few minutes. Make sure that the texture and softness of the broccoli is not hindered.

Drain the broccoli and set it aside so that the steam evaporates from it.

Grease a baking dish and arrange the broccoli on it and season it with butter and pepper, according to your taste. Sprinkle the grated cheddar cheese on broccoli and bake it for 15-20 minutes. Make sure that the cheese turns golden as it portrays that the dish is ready.

While the broccoli is being baked, season the salmon with salt and pepper. Fry it in butter for a good few minutes on both sides. You can fry the lime along the salmon or leave it out if you want to. Arrange all the elements on a plate and you have a scrumptious meal ready to be gulped!

Day 10:
Wednesday:

- **Breakfast: Keto Coconut Porridge:**

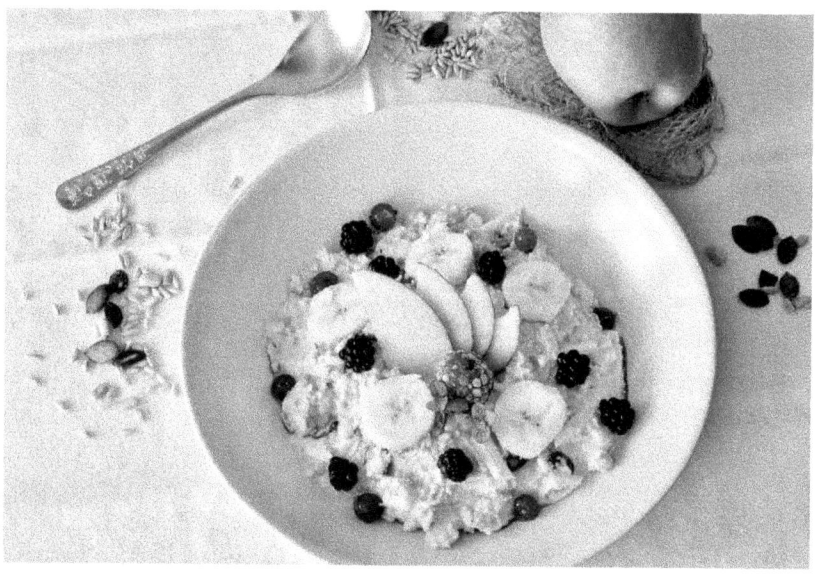

Are you looking forward to a hot cereal dish this morning? This is a very comfortable and satisfying meal, for your belly! A very pure and glee filled breakfast meal it is.

Ingredients:

You will need:

- Coconut-1 oz.
- Egg-1

- Coconut flour-1 tbsp.
- Coconut cream-4 tbsp.
- Salt- 1 pinch
- Ground psyllium husk powder-1 pinch

Preparation:

Add all the ingredients in a non-stick pan and mix them together on low flame. Stir continually until you get the perfect texture that you want.

Serve it all with coconut cream or milk. You can also top the cereal with berries.

- **Lunch: Keto shrimp and artichoke plate:**

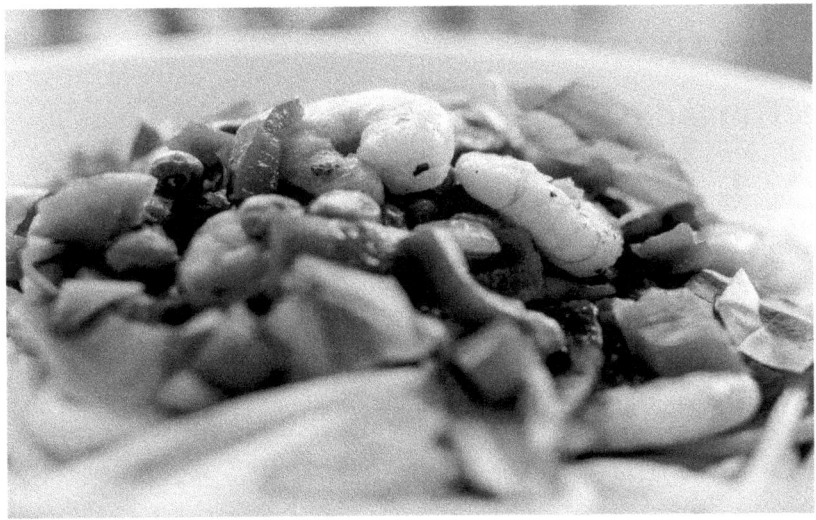

This lunch meal is all you need for having real food on plate. Simple and free of complications, this meal is very quick and easy to make.

- **Dinner: Keto Chicken Casserole:**

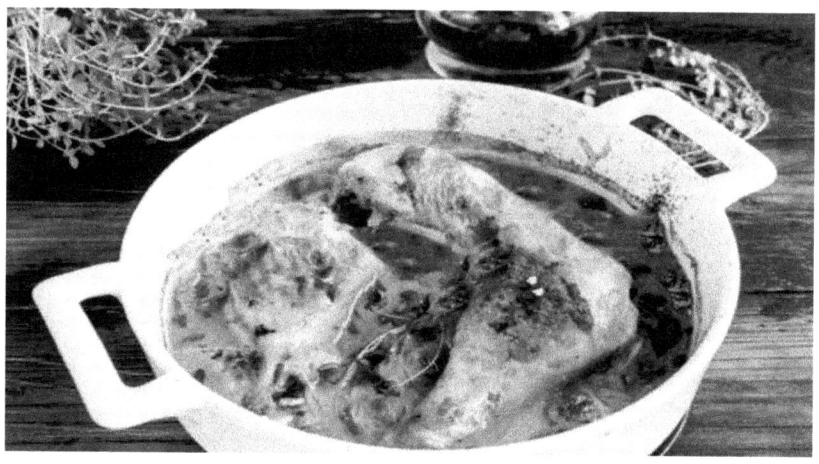

This casserole is the best keto meal for all the dieters. The cheesy and creamy sauce is the perfect punch of flavors that anyone would wish for.

Day 11:
Thursday:

- **Breakfast: Keto Egg Muffins:**

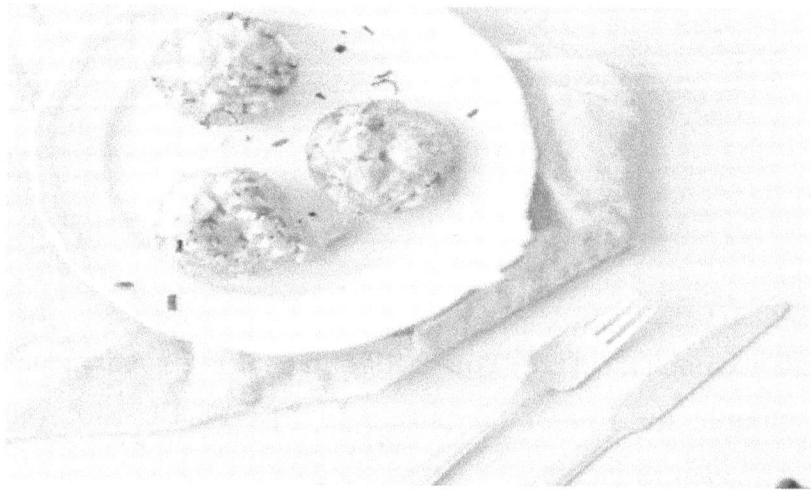

Keto egg muffins are highly time saving and are super convenient to make. You can make them ahead of time and enjoy a lot.

- **Lunch: Keto Cauliflower Soup with crumbled pancetta:**

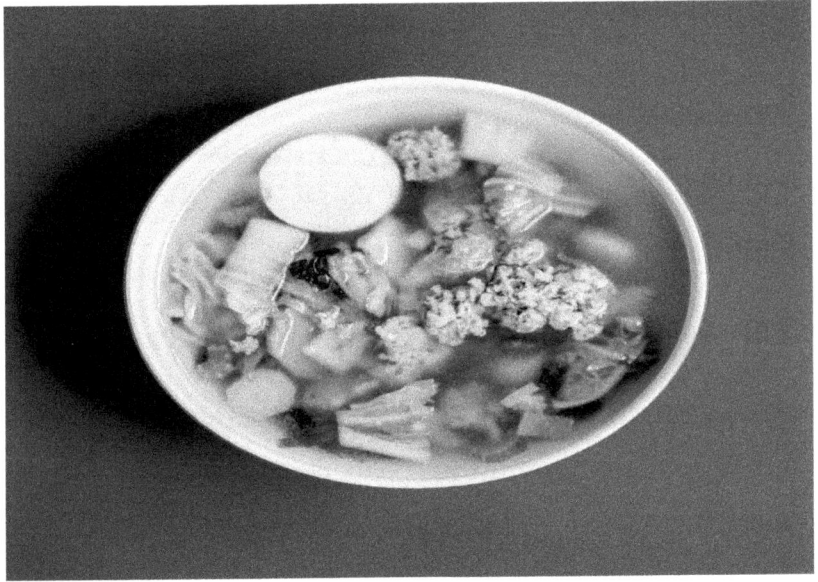

This cauliflower soup is quick to make and is super satisfying too. Creamy soup, with a healthy topping of fried pancetta and nuts and cauliflower is the perfect keto lunch for all the dieters out there. Very luxurious and yummy!

Ingredients:

You will need:

- Chicken broth or vegetable stock-4 cups

- Cream cheese-7 oz.
- Butter-4 oz.
- Salt and Pepper
- Dijon mustard-1 tbsp.
- Pancetta (diced)-7 oz.
- Butter for frying-1 tbsp.
- Pecans-3 oz.
- Paprika Powder-1 tsp.

Preparation:

Cut the cauliflower in small pieces. Tip; the smaller the cauliflower, the faster the soup is ready.

Put aside some cauliflower and cut into ¼ inch pieces.

Sautee the pancetta and cauliflower together and once they are crispy; add the nuts and paprika powder to it. Mix well and set it aside.

Boil the cauliflower pieces in the stock until they get soft. Then add butter, cream cheese and Dijon mustard to it. Now, with the help of an immersion blender, mix the soup to get the texture or consistency that you want. The creamier you want the soup to be; the more you blend it. Season it with salt and pepper, according to your taste.

Pour the soup in the bowls and top it with fried pancetta mix.

- **Dinner: Keto Cheeseburger:**

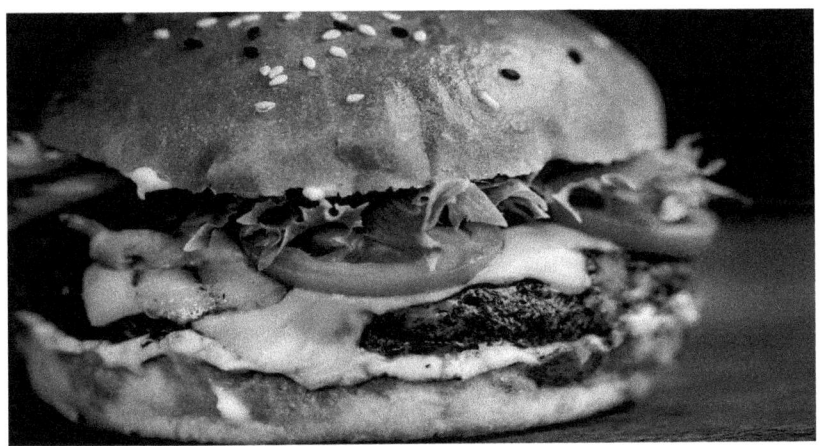

Keto cheeseburger is a very casual feast but extremely delicious too. It is satisfying and has a punch of flavor and is extremely light for dinner too.

Day 12:
Friday:

- **Breakfast: Boiled Eggs with Mayonnaise:**

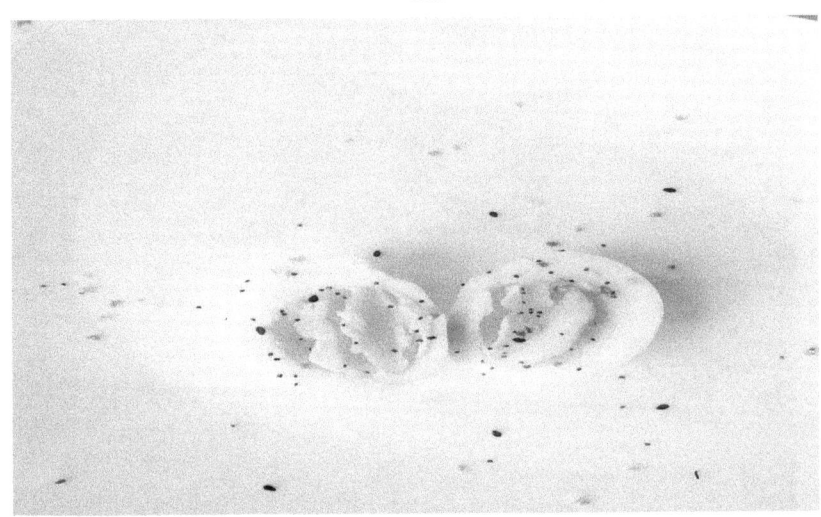

This is for all the egg lovers who want simplicity in their meal. It is very quick to make and is fully satisfying for the tummy too.

- **Lunch: Keto Caesar Salad:**

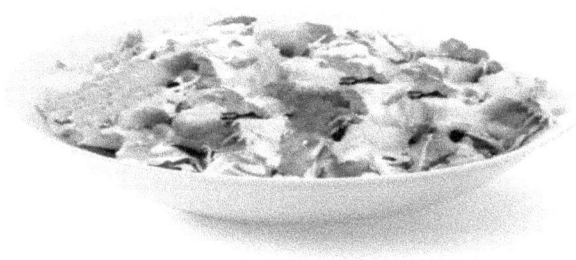

Keto Caesar salad is a perfect keto classic that every dieter will fall in love with.

- **Dinner: Fathead Pizza:**

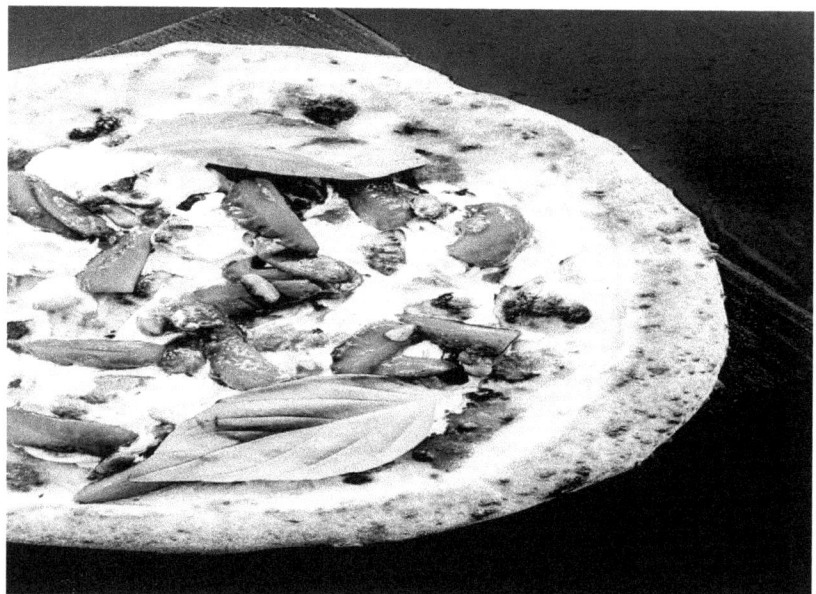

Fathead pizza is satisfying and mouthwatering and has the perfect crunchy and cheesy feel to it! Here's how you can make it to have the best dinner.

Ingredients:

You will need:

- For the topping:
- Butter- 1 tbsp.
- Unsweetened tomato sauce- ½ cup
- Dried Oregano- ½ tsp
- Shredded mozzarella cheese- 4 ½ oz.
- Fresh Italian Sausage-8 oz.
- For the crust:
- White wine vinegar-1 tsp.
- Egg-1
- Salt- ½ tsp.
- Olive oil for greasing your hands
- Almond Flour- ¾ cup
- Cream Cheese-2 tbsp.
- Shredded ozzarella Cheese-

Preparation:

Preheat the oven at 200 degree Celsius.

Meanwhile, heat the cream cheese and mozzarella in a pan, on medium flame. Stir both of them constantly so that they mix really well together. Once they have combined, mix all the other ingredients in it.

Once ready, apply olive oil on your hands and spread the dough out on a parchment paper. Flatten it and then prick the dough with the help of a fork. Place it in the oven for 10-15 minutes. Make sure that it turns slightly golden brown and the remove from the oven.

While the dough is being baked, melt butter or heat olive oil and sauté the ground beef or meat in it. Once the crust is done, spread a little tomato sauce on it and top it with meat and loads of cheese. Place it back in the oven at bake for around 10-15 minutes.

Sprinkle a little oregano on top and enjoy a scrumptious meal!

Day 13:
Saturday:

- **Breakfast: Western Omelet Breakfast:**

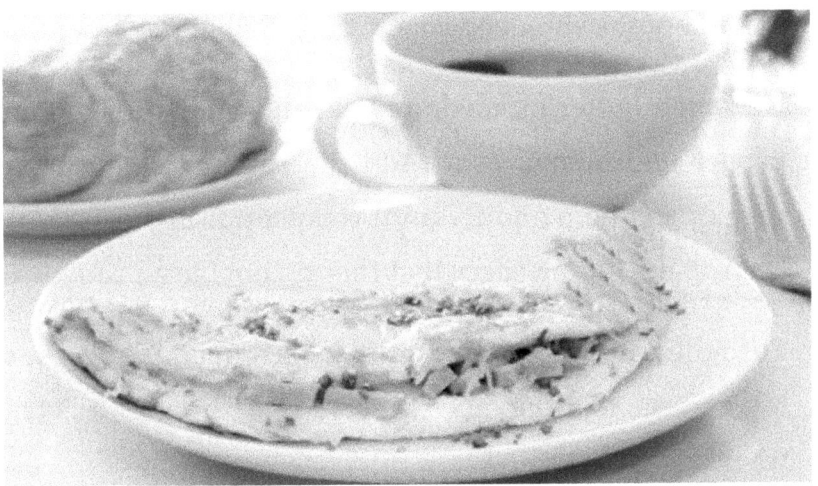

Packed with goodness of cheese and eggs, this fluffy omelet is everything that you might need and crave for a perfect breakfast, on Saturday morning.

Ingredients:

You will need:

- Eggs-6
- Heavy whipping cream-2 tbsp.
- Shredded Cheese- 3 oz.
- Salt and pepper
- Butter-2 oz.
- Diced, smoked deli ham-5 oz.
- Finely chopped, green bell pepper- 1/2
- Finely chopped yellow onion- 1/2

Preparation:

Whisk together eggs and whipping cream until they are fluffy and then add salt and pepper to it. Further add half amount of the shredded cheese and combine well.

Now melt butter on medium heat and sauté the ham, bell pepper and onions in it. Add the egg and cream to the veggies and ham and fry until you get a firm omelet. Also, keep an eye on the edges that they do not burn.

Turn the flame to low and sprinkle the remaining cheese on top and the fold the omelet. Serve right away as it is tasty when served hot.

- **Lunch: Keto prosciutto-wrapped asparagus with goat cheese:**

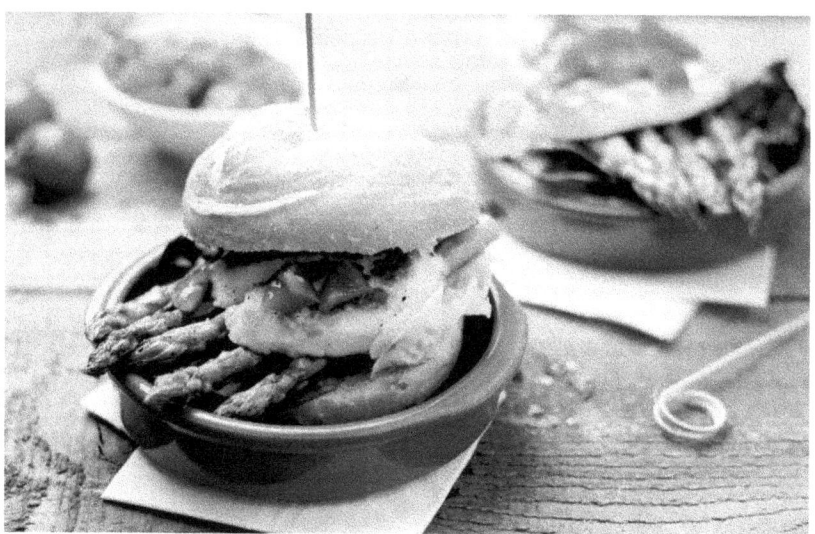

This is the perfect trio of flavors that any keto dieter would want. It is very easy to make and is definitely an elegant dish to serve to you.

- **Dinner: Creamy Keto Fish Casserole:**

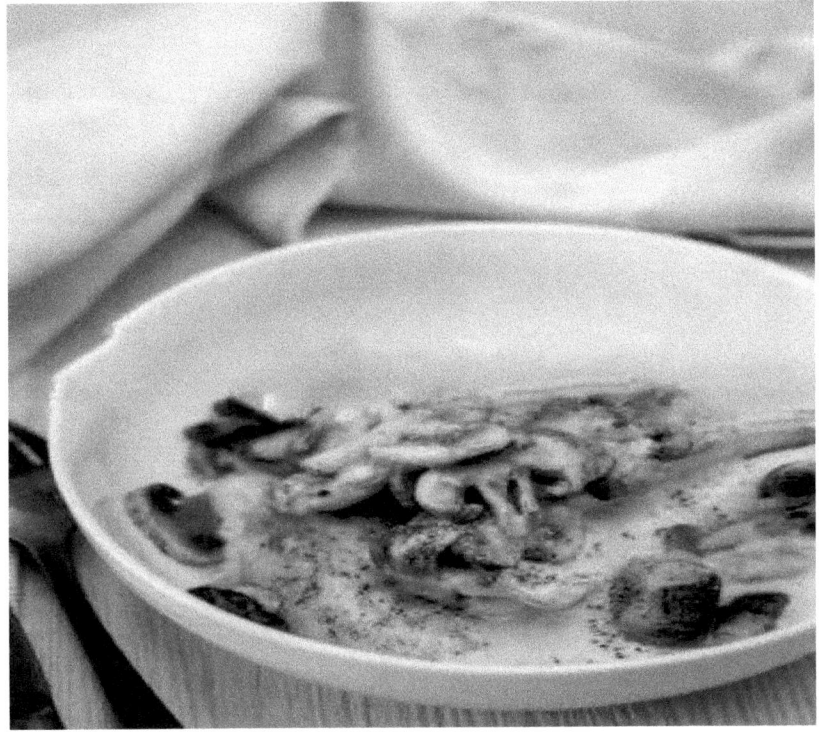

Creamy gravy with fish in it is the best dinner that you would want. A perfect blend of flavors makes this dish one of the best dinners and is super easy to make too.

Day 14:
Sunday:

- **Breakfast: Classic Bacon and Eggs:**

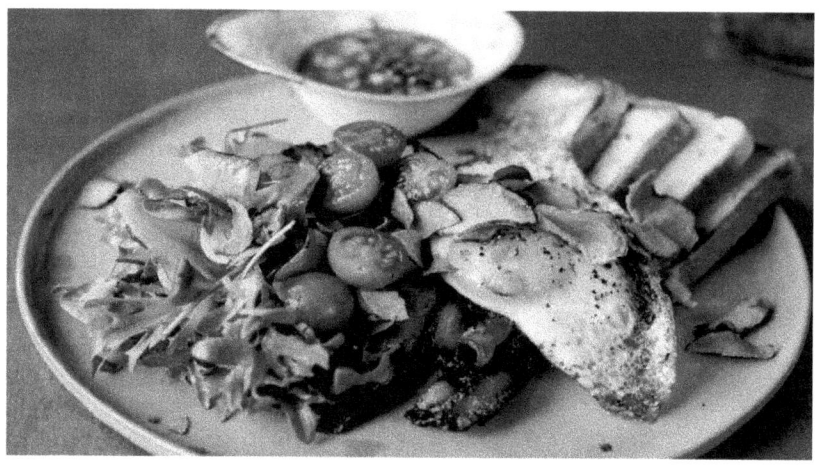

Classic bacon and eggs is an all time winner to opt for as a keto breakfast. it is extremely mouthwatering and is the best breakfast that gives you the right punch of energy in the morning.

- **Lunch: Keto Salmon filled Avocados:**

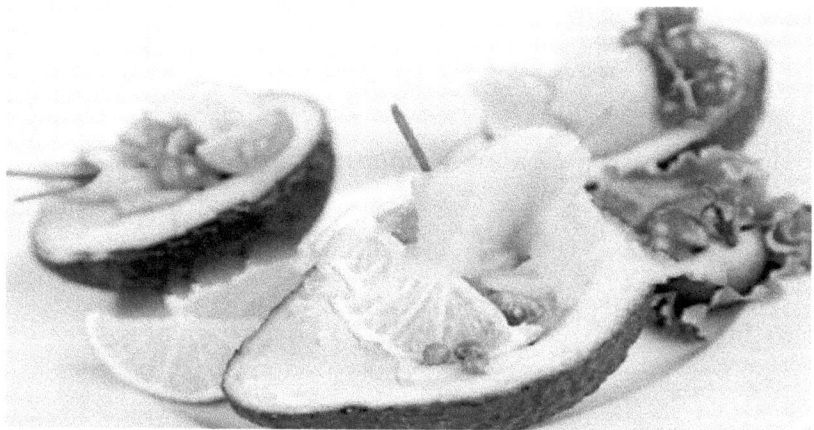

This combination of avocados and salmon brings you a simple to make meal which requires no cooking. It is a wonderful lunch meal and can be served as dinner too as it is very light.

Ingredients:

You will need:

- Smoked Salmon-6 oz.
- Salt and pepper
- Sour cream-3/4 cup
- Avocados-2
- Lemon juice-2 tbsp. (optional)

Preparation:

Remove the pit from the avocados and cut them in half.

Put sour cream in the hollow of the avocados (you can also use mayonnaise) and top it with salmon. Season with salt and pepper and a little lemon if you would like and the meal is all ready to eat!

- **Dinner: Keto Ribeye Steak with oven-roasted vegetables:**

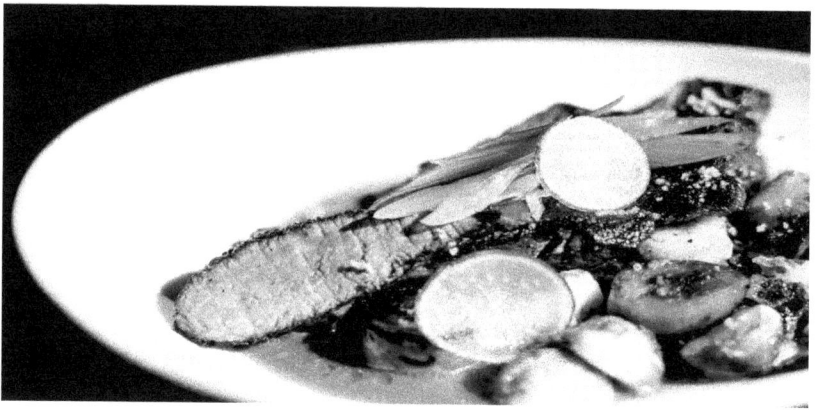

Nothing is more eye catching than a ribeye steak which is seasoned with anchovy butter. Really easy and quick to make; it is a dinner worth a Sunday evening.

Week 3

Day 15:

Monday:

- **Breakfast: Keto Avocado Eggs with Bacon Sails:**

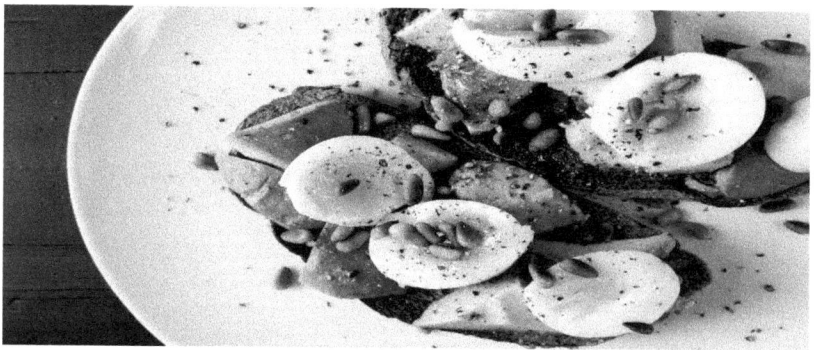

This is a wonderful breakfast twist that everyone keto dieter will admire. It tastes heavenly and will make you want to get out of bed earlier. This is perfect for a Monday morning to beat down the blues.

- **Lunch: Diary Free Butter Chicken:**

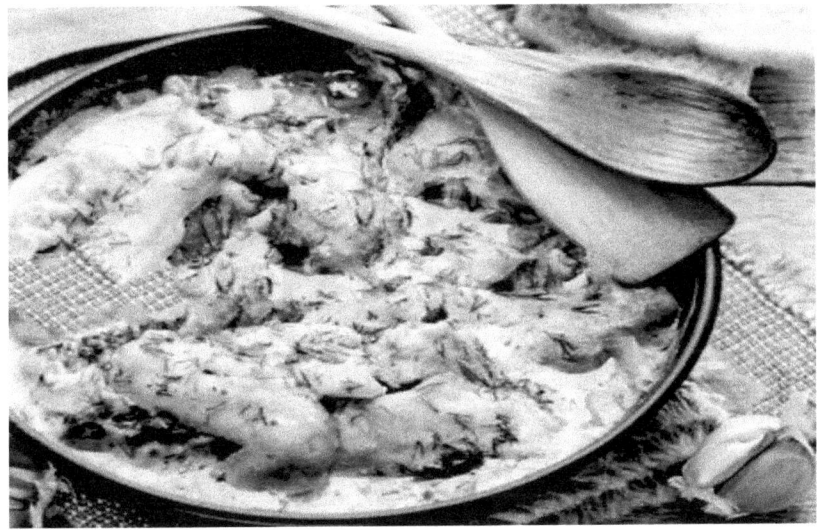

The keto butter chicken just has 7 net carbs which is the perfect dish to have at a Monday noon. Pack it up at work and you can have it with raw vegetables or cauliflower rice too.

- **Dinner: Salad Sandwiches**

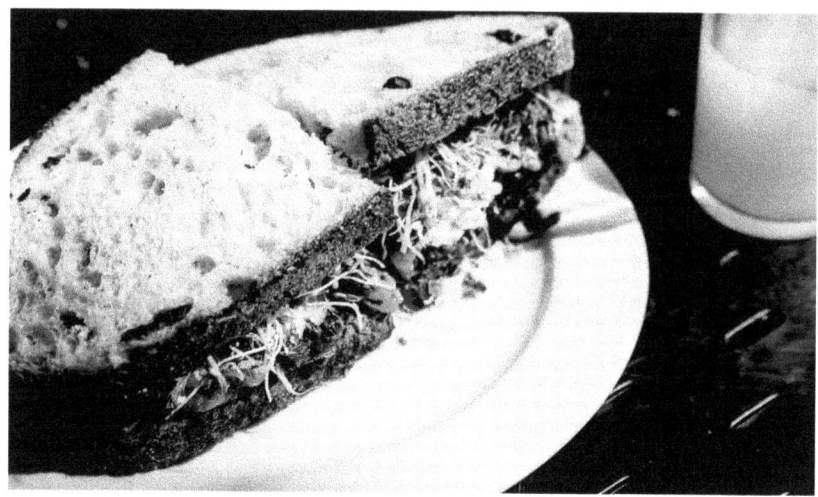

Being on keto doesn't mean that you have to say goodbye to your sandwiches. You can make one without bread too and it tastes nothing but wonderful.

Ingredients:

You will need:

- Romaine lettuce-2 oz.
- Cherry tomatoes-1
- Avocado-1/2
- Butter-1/2 oz
- Edam cheese-1 oz.

Preparation:

Clean the lettuce thoroughly and make it the base of your sandwich. Smear a little butter on the lettuce leaves and add sliced tomatoes, cheese and avocado on top. It is as simple as this and your dinner is ready with this quick meal.

Day 16:
Tuesday:

- **Breakfast: Keto Tuna Salad with Capers:**

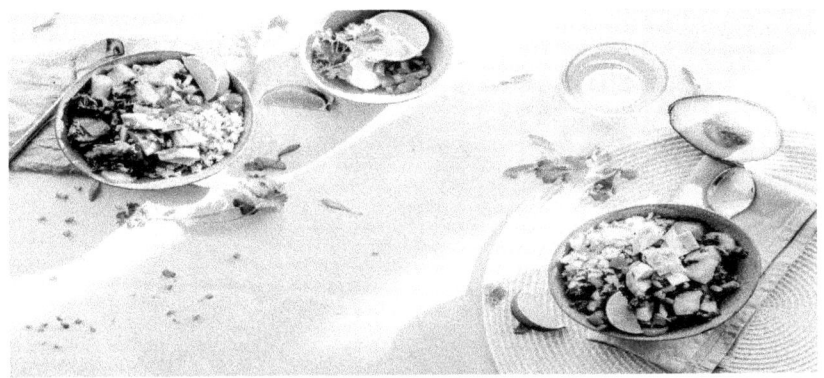

This tuna salad crosses the boundaries of an ordinary salad and is very classic and yummy.

Ingredients:

You will need:

- Tuna in Olive oil-4 oz.
- Mayonnaise- 1/2 cup
- Capers-1 tbsp.
- Salt and pepper
- Chili flakes-1/2 tsp
- Finely chopped leek-1/2
- Capers-1/2
- Crème Fraiche-2 tbsp.

Preparation:

Drain the tuna and mix all the ingredients together. Combine them well and season them with chili flakes, salt and pepper. And that is it! Serve alongside boiled eggs and you will love your breakfast.

- **Lunch: Bacon Spinach Frittata:**

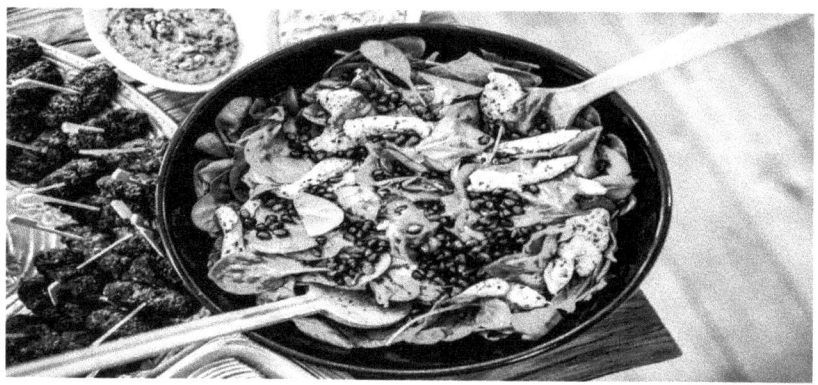

This lunch recipe has just 6.5 net carbs and can be enjoyed hot and cold both. Baked eggs are the perfect base for bacon and spinach. You can also use any other vegetable that you might have at your right hand access and make this delicious lunch.

- **Dinner: Low Carb Taco Pie:**

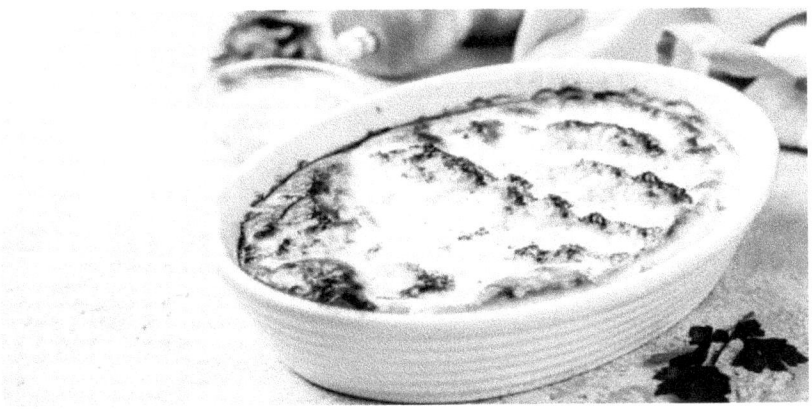

Taco pie is very easy to make and has all the flavors that one would want for a dinner meal. It sums up for a perfect dinner and you won't regret making it!

Day 17:
Wednesday:

- **Breakfast: Breakfast Tapas:**

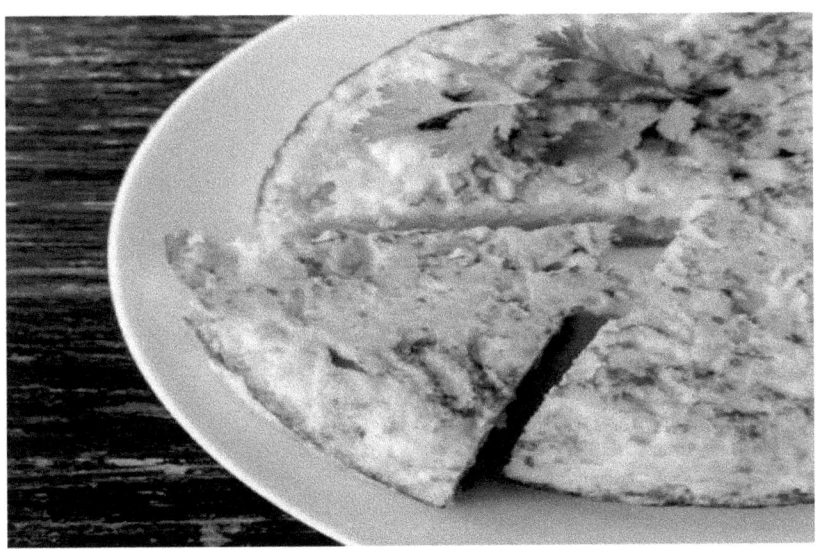

Breakfast tapas are the show stealer and very simple to make. A powerful combination of cheeses, veggies and nuts is all that makes it a power pack breakfast dish.

- **Lunch: Keto Turkey with Cream Cheese Sauce:**

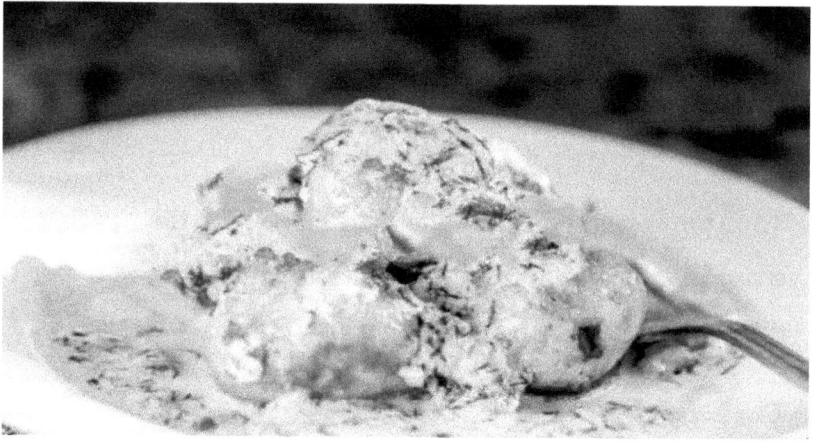

This meal's simplicity is the show stealer and has a power of flavors that will make you fall in love with this dish. Satisfying and succulent are the perfect words to describe it.

Ingredients:

You will need:

- Butter-2 tbsp.
- Turkey breast-20 oz.
- Crèmefraiche or heavy whipping cream- 2 cups
- Cream cheese-7 oz.

- Salt and pepper
- Small capers- 1/3 cup
- Tamari soy sauce- 1 tbsp.

Preparation:

Preheat the oven at 170 degree Celsius.

Meanwhile, melt half of the butter on medium flame and season the turkey according to your tastes. Fry it until it is golden brown.

Place the turkey in the oven to finish it off properly. The timing will depend and you will have to check on the turkey again and again. Once done, take it out on a plate and tent it with foil.

Take the drippings of the turkey in a saucepan and add sour cream and cream cheese to it. Stir it and let it boil a bit. Lower down the flame and allow it to simmer until it has thickened. Season a bit with salt and pepper.

Now melt the remaining butter in another pan and sauté the capers in it until they are crispy. Serve the turkey with the capers and sauce and have the best lunch ever.

- **Dinner: Chops Marinated in Red Pesto:**

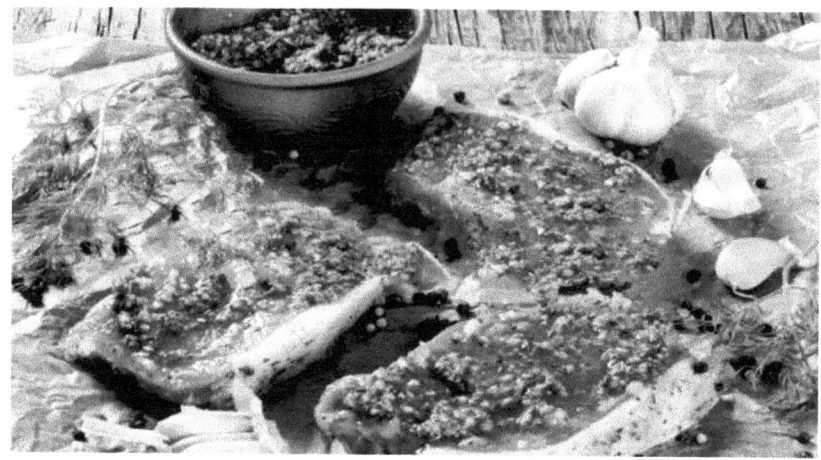

This dinner meal has just 1g net carb and is very easy and quick to make. Fix a wonderfully tasty dinner for yourself within no time and have fun.

Day 18:
Thursday:

- **Breakfast: Fried Eggs:**

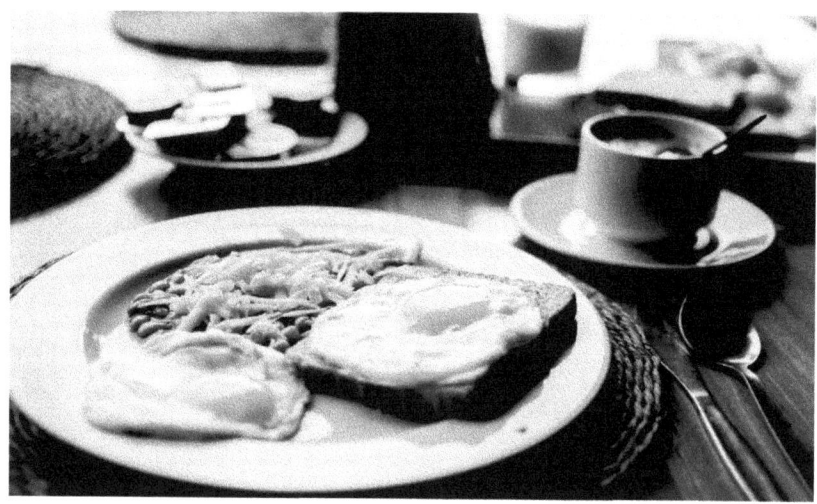

Fried eggs are a pleasure for life and you can enjoy the best fried eggs on keto diet too. Get yourself the best fried egg keto recipe and you can have your style eggs in the morning.

- **Lunch: Bison Meatballs with Zoodles and Chimichurri Sauce:**

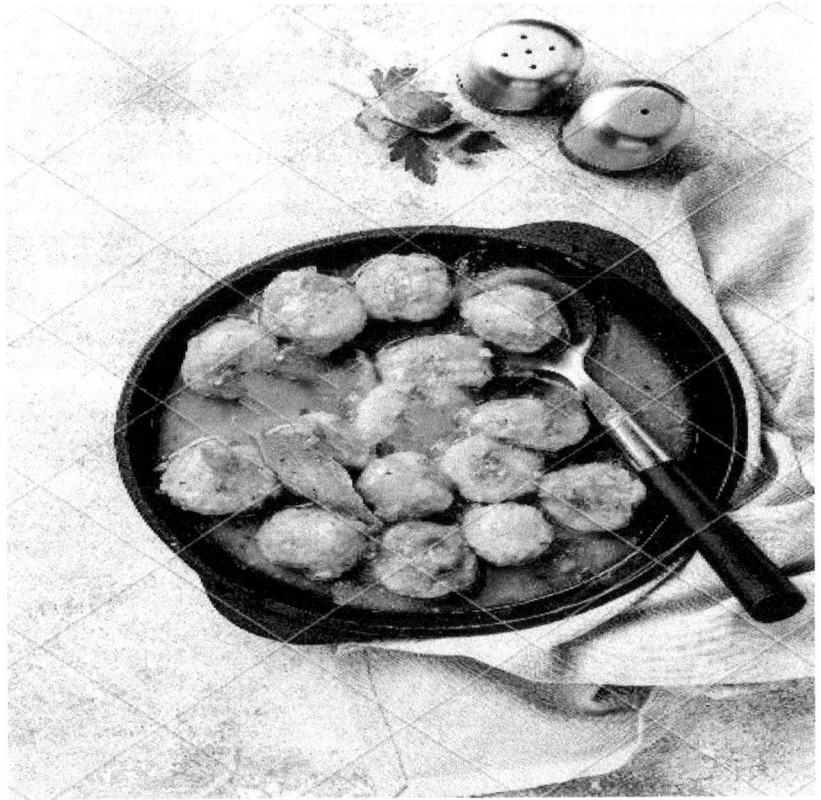

The perfect meatballs with a herb infused sauce is the perfect combination of flavors that one needs during lunch. It has just 6.6g net carbs which leaves a lot of carb limit for you, for your dinner.

- **Dinner: Keto baked Salmon with Pesto:**

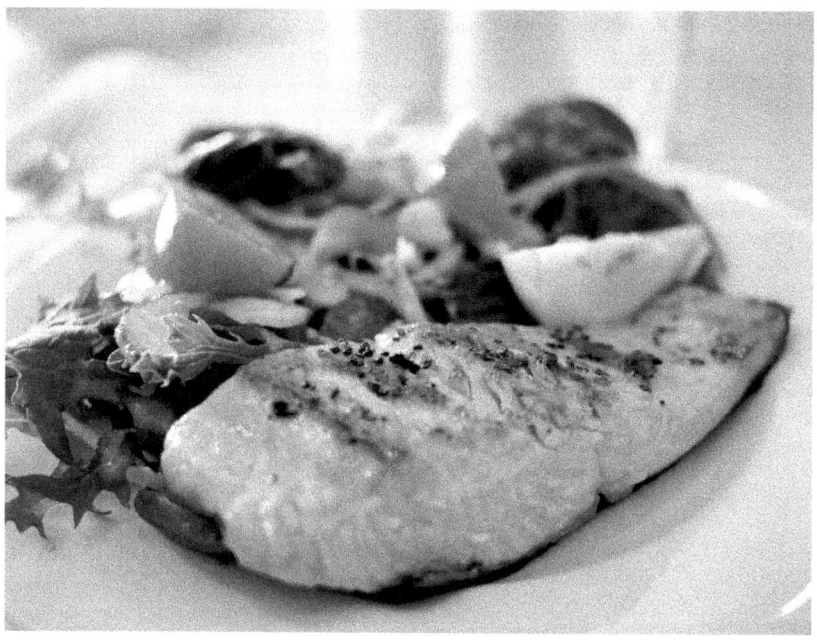

This baked salmon with pesto is the simplest meal that one needs on a tiring and hectic day. It is easy to make and taste wonderful.

Ingredients:

You will need:

- Green Pesto-2 oz.
- Salt and Pepper
- Mayonnaise-1 cup
- Greek Yogurt-1/2 cup
- Salmon-30 oz.
- Green Pesto-2 oz.

Preparation:

Grease the baking dish and place the salmon, upside down on it. Spread pesto on it and season with salt and pepper. Bake in oven at 200 degree Celsius and for around 30 minutes. The salmon should flake easily with a fork.

Stir together green pesto, mayonnaise and Greek yogurt to create a sauce and serve it along with baked salmon.

Day 19:
Friday:

- **Breakfast: Scrambled Egg with Basil and Butter:**

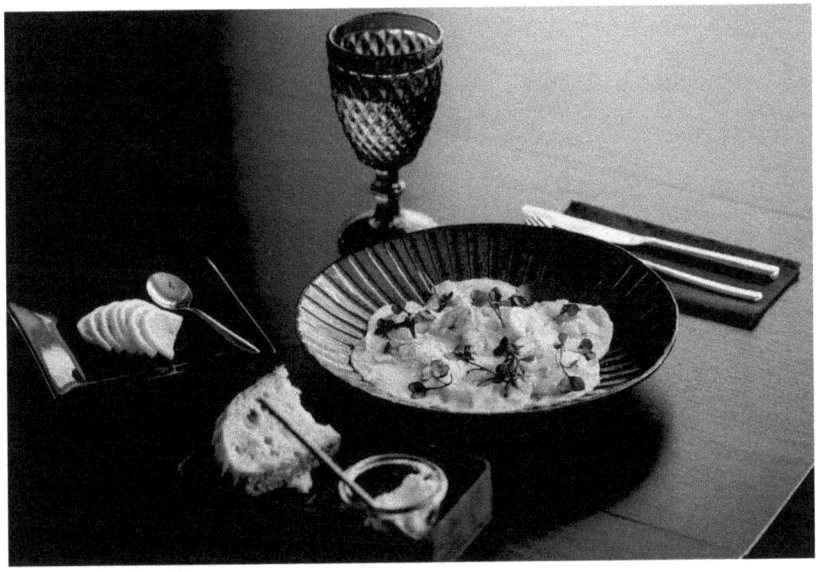

This is a very classical and wonderfully dressed up breakfast meal which gives you the right herbs and combo of egg and butter to bring the satisfying feeling too.

Ingredients:

You will need:

- Eggs-2
- coconut cream or coconut milk or sour cream-2 tbsp.
- salt
- butter-1 oz.
- shredded cheese (optional)
- fresh basil-2 tbsp

Preparation:

Melt butter on low heat and meanwhile, whisk eggs, cream and salt in a small bowl. Add it to the pan, in the melted butter. Stir it in the center of the pan and until the eggs are scrambled and make sure that they are not too crispy. Soft and creamy scrambled are the best. Once done, top it with a little fresh basil and you are good to go.

- **Lunch: California Turkey and Bacon Wraps with Basil Mayo:**

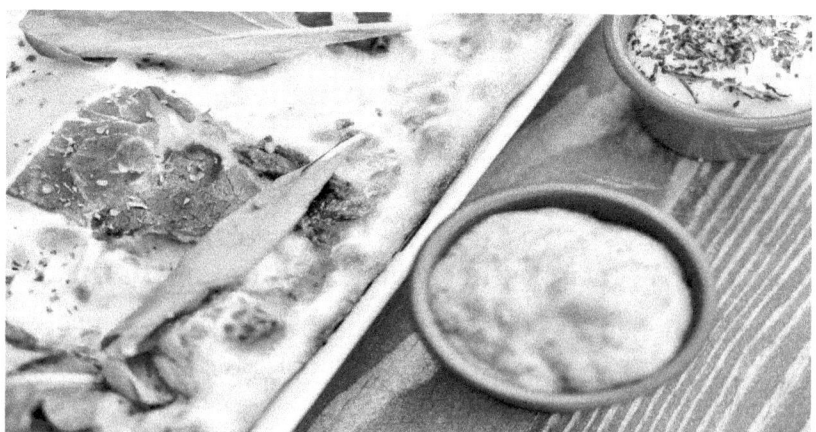

These wraps are fresh and satisfying and make a wonderful lunch meal! Low in carbs, this turkey and bacon wrap is going to be your best lunch!

- **Dinner: Keto Meatballs:**

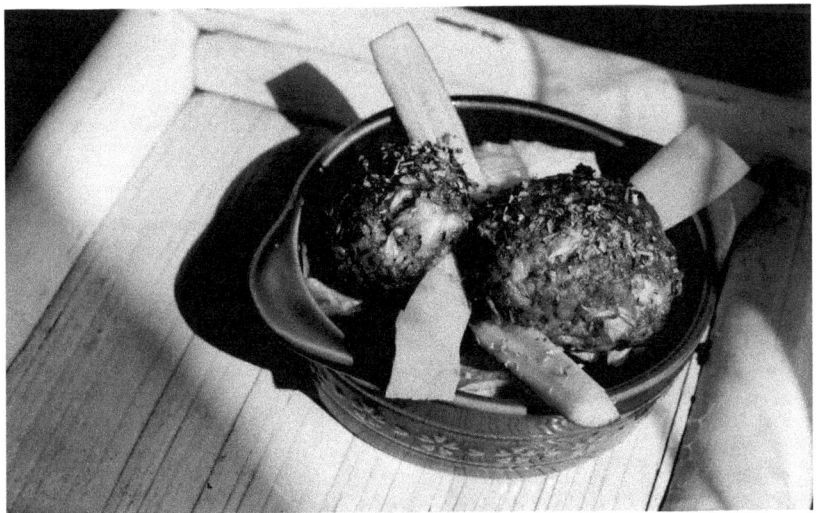

- Skip the flour as these meatballs are all about healthy fat, in which cheese holds them together, providing a great rush of taste in your mouth. This is a whiff of fresh air in the world of keto dieters and you are definitely going to love it.

Day 20:

Saturday:

- **Breakfast: Keto Cauliflower Hash with Eggs and Poblano Peppers:**

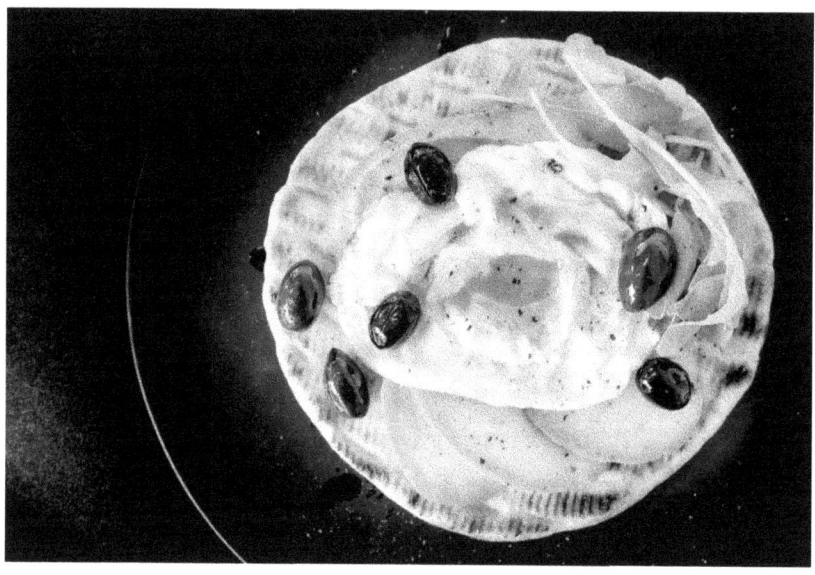

This is a punch of southwest flavors, combined with eggs and potatoes. It is a sophisticated dish which makes a powerful breakfast and offers out a satisfying feeling in the morning.

- **Lunch: Blackened Shrimp, Asparagus and Avocado Salad:**

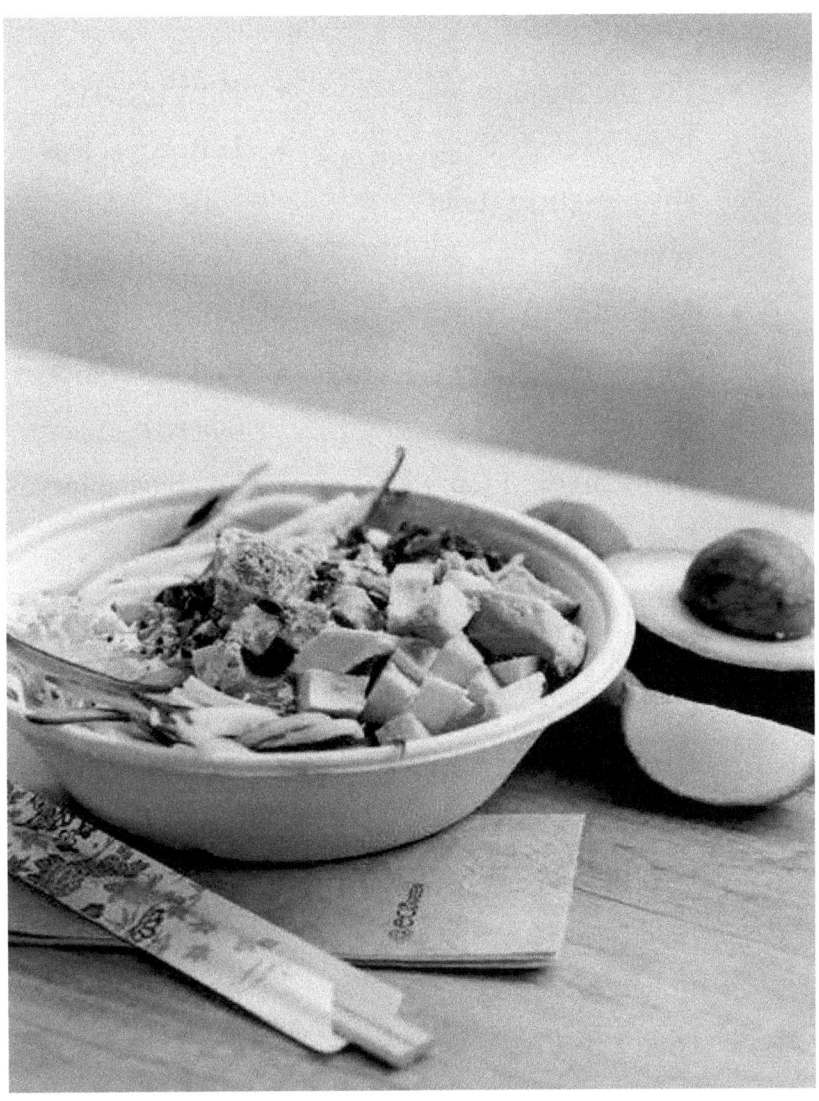

This is the perfect keto salad, which is ready to eat within 10 minutes and tastes heavenly too. Here is how you can make it;

Ingredients:

You will need:

- For the Shrimp:
- Raw peeled large shrimp-500 g (tails removed)
- Minced garlic-2 cloves
- Ground basil- 1 tsp.
- Dried thyme-1 tsp.
- Sea salt-1 tsp.
- Fresh cracked black pepper-1 tsp.
- Cayenne pepper-1 tsp.
- Sweet paprika-2 tsps.
- Asparagus-2 (cut in halves)
- Olive oil- 1 tsp.

- For the Salad:
- Lettuce leaves-4 cups
- Avocado-1 (cut in cubes)
- Red onion-1/4 (sliced)
- Fresh basil leaves-1 handful
- For the dressing:
- Greek yogurt-1/3 cup
- Lemon pepper-1 tsp.
- Lemon juice-1 tsp. 9optional)
- Water-2 tbsp.
- Salt to taste

Preparation:

Take a good sized bowl and mix all the shrimp ingredients together. Make sure that you rub the spices on all shrimps so that they enhance the taste that you require. Heat olive oil in a large skillet and sauté the marinated shrimps in it, along with asparagus. Toss and turn them time to time until the shrimps have changed their color and are cooked. This will take around 5 minutes.

Now, in a salad bowl, combine all the salad ingredients and add the cooked shrimps and asparagus on top of it. Whisk the dressing ingredients in a separate bowl and pour it over the salad and enjoy your meal!

- **Dinner: Keto Bacon Sushi:**

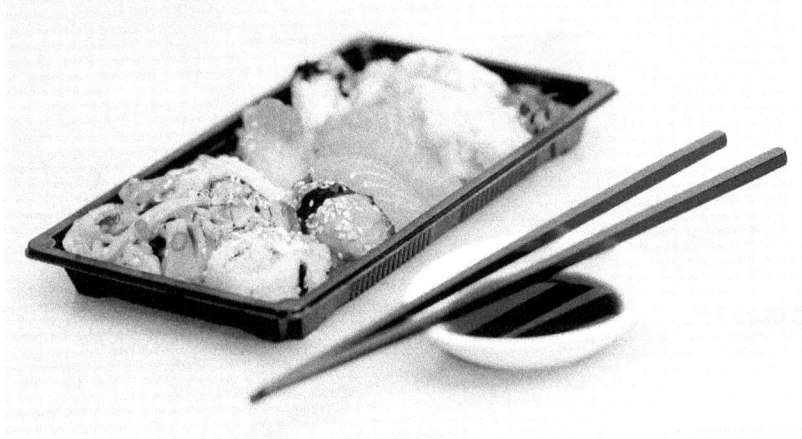

These tiny little bacon sushi wraps are the most satisfying pieces of heaven for all the keto dieters and the sushi lovers too. They are a perfect combo of crunchy, salty and creamy!

Day 21:

Sunday:

- **Breakfast: Keto Fried Eggs with Kale and Pork:**

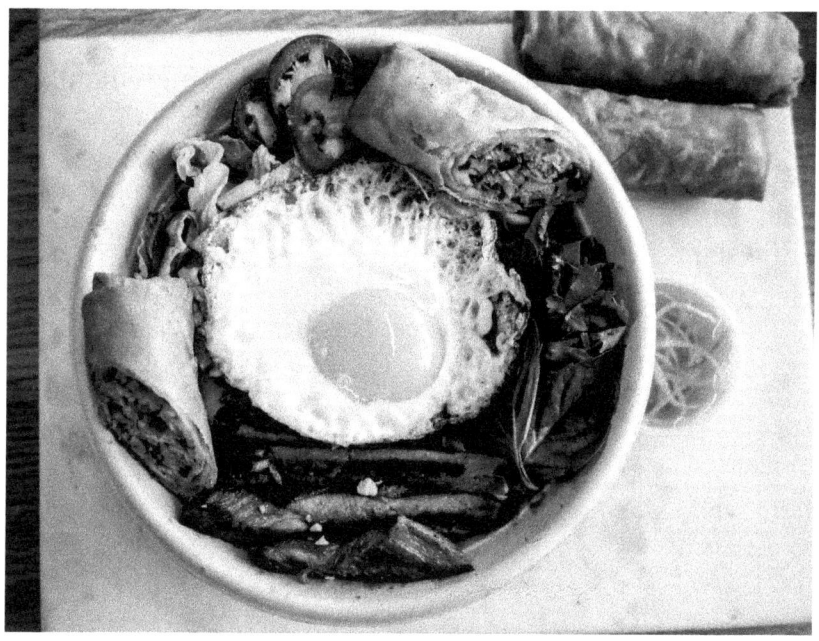

Bring it on! This delicious combination of eggs and veggies with the perfect crispiness of pork is all you want for a wonderful Sunday morning meal. Quick to make and quicker to gulp down!

- **Lunch: Salad with Roasted Cauliflower:**

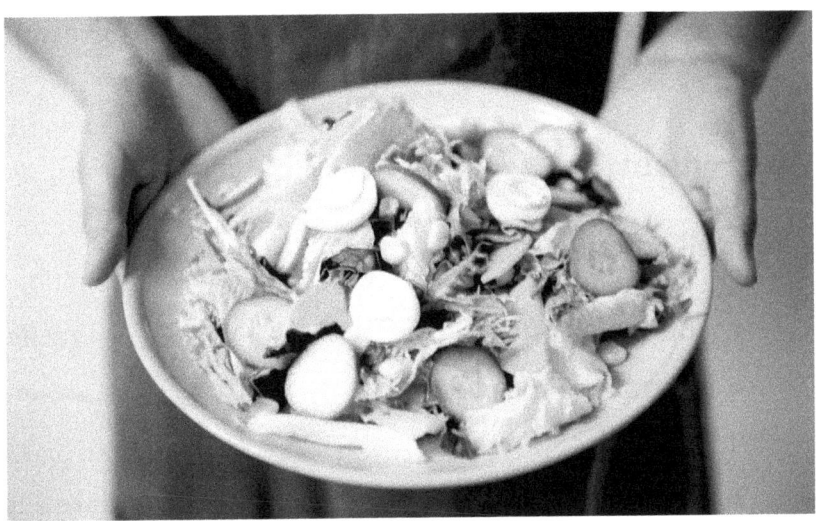

If you are a vegan, keto is not that hard though! Recipes like these are the perfect example of how wonderful ketosis can be for vegans. It has healthy fats which makes this dish heavily satisfying and delicious.

- **Dinner: Garlicky Lemon Mahi-Mahi:**

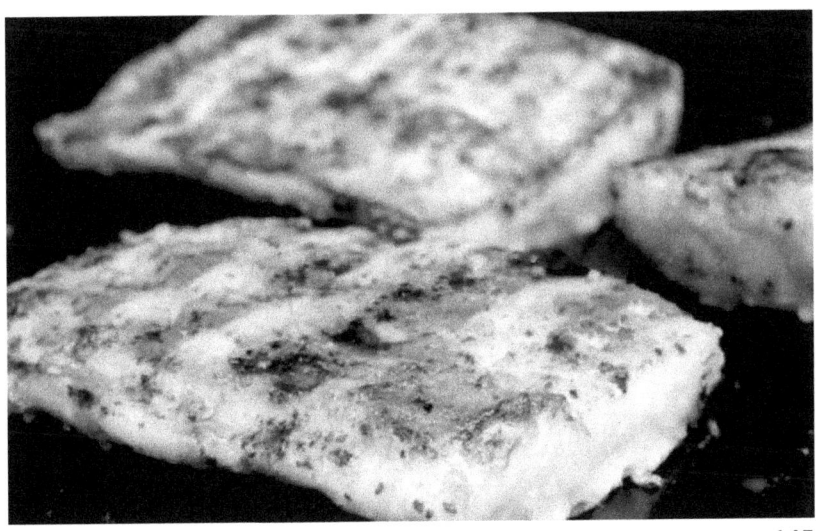

The name of the dish is certainly different and so is its taste! This is a great, 30 minutes dish which fulfills your protein cravings just right.

Ingredients:

You will need:

- Butter-3 tbsp.
- Extra-virgin olive oil-2 tbsp.
- Mahi-mahi fillets-4 oz.
- Kosher salt
- Freshly ground black pepper
- Asparagus-1 lb.
- Minced garlic-1 clove
- Crushed red pepper flakes-1/4 tsp.
- Lemon-1 (sliced)
- Zest and juice lemon-1
- Freshly chopped parsley-1 tbsp.

Preparation:

Melt 1 tbsp. of butter and 1 tbsp. of olive oil in a skillet, over medium flame and add mahi-mahi fillets to it. Season it with salt and pepper and cook it until golden. It is going to require 4-5 minutes on each side; so don't rush.

Once done, remove the fillets on a plate and add asparagus to the same skillet. Cook for around 2-3 minutes until it is tender and season it with salt and pepper too. Once done, remove the asparagus in a plate too.

Now add the remaining tbsp. butter to the skillet and melt it. Then add garlic and red pepper flakes to it. Sauté them for a minute and then add lemon zest, juice and parsley. Stir it properly. Once done, add the mahi-mahi and asparagus to the skillet and garnish it with the dressing. Serve hot and enjoy your Sunday dinner to the fullest.

This is a complete 21 day meal plan for keto which will help you have limited carbs, good and healthy fats along with moderate protein intake, without crossing any restrictions. You can get taste and health both with these delicious recipes. Stop believing people who tell you that ketosis is not good for your taste buds. If you invest a little time, these meals are way healthier and yummier than your old ones.

Self-care Tips for Transition in Ketosis Intermittent Fasting:

Important Minerals and Vitamins during Ketosis:
There is simply no doubt that ketogenic diet is a completely normal metabolic state. However, there are still some deficiencies that a person does face during keto or intermittent fasting. It is always a good idea to take the important mineral and nutrients through supplements while you are on ketosis or else, you can face trouble with

your body deficiencies. If done correctly, keto dieters usually don't face a lot of problems or deficiencies but people usually go to extremes with this diet plan and then find their bodies giving up to the entire program. This is where; some vitamin and mineral supplements can be helpful.

Here is a list of important mineral and vitamins that every human body needs. If you are keto dieter, make sure that you are taking them in adequate amount:

- **Sodium:** In a low carb diet, your body needs sodium so that it can fight against headaches and fatigue. Until and unless you have a medical issue that states your low sodium intake; it is safe to take around 3000mg of sodium per day. There are various sources through which you can take sodium, like, bone broth, adding sea vegetables to your diet or using sea salt in your food.

- **Potassium:** Potassium is a very crucial element for the human body and one must take care of it, during ketogenic diet. 2000mg potassium per day, for a keto dieter, is sufficient and recommended too. It is best that you do not consume potassium supplements as they are toxic. You can easily gain it through avocados, salmon, mushrooms, green veggies and nuts.

- **Magnesium:** Magnesium is yet another important element for the human body as it keeps the energy system running efficiently. Sadly, majority of people have low magnesium levels and they are not aware of it either. While on ketosis, you can easily run out of proper magnesium thus it is important that you take a supplement for it. Consulting your nutritionist or doctor will definitely be recommended in this case.

- **Calcium:** Calcium can be flushed out of the human body while it is settling into the ketosis phase and running around without good amount of calcium is somewhat impossible. Diary is the most common source of calcium but it is restricted during ketogenic diet. However, broccoli, fish, kale and unsweetened almond milk are also great sources for attaining calcium. However, if you still think that your body has low calcium levels, then you can consult your doctor and get calcium supplements.

How to work out while on Ketogenic Fasting?

A lot of people doubt exercising while they are fasting. The doubt is definitely solid because working out while you are on an intermittent fast, does have its cons. There are certainly a lot of perks too but the negative impact is also there.

A lot of researches state that exercising while you are fasting can actually be very healthy and helpful for your metabolism and can also boost stability in blood sugar levels. Even though this does sound amazing because your body will be burning fat rapidly but there is a huge downfall too. You won't be able to work out with a lot of power. A 30 minute workout might just end within 10 minutes because you will run short of energy sooner. Also, a lot of nutritionists do not recommended working out while fasting. You are already low on calories and carbs and this can lead to several deficiencies. It is best to work out during the 8 hour window because you are actually providing your body with the nutrients, vitamins and minerals and exercising won't make you fall short of them.

Therefore, it is highly recommended that you do not work out while you are fasting. And if you do have to, keep it extremely short and don't try to attempt heavy weight lifting or high intensity training.

www.ingramcontent.com/pod-product-compliance
Ingram Content Group UK Ltd.
Pitfield, Milton Keynes, MK11 3LW, UK
UKHW022225230426
12048UKWH00016BA/1074